Rapid Weight Loss Hypnosis Mastery

2 Books in 1

The Ultimate Subliminal Affirmations to Naturally Lose Weight, Feel Healthy and Quit Sugar & Stop Sugar Cravings, & to Love Your Body

Written By

DAVID JENKINS

Table of Contents

Hypnosis and Meditation for Weight Loss

Table of Contents

Weight Loss Hypnosis Mastery

Hypnosis and Meditation for Weight Loss

The Ultimate Subliminal Affirmations to Naturally Lose Weight, Feel Healthy and with Self-Hypnosis, Meditation and Affirmation

Written By

DAVID JENKINS

INTRODUCTION

Thank you for purchasing this book!

A non-pharmacological way to improve sleep is hypnosis. Although there are different definitions of hypnosis, Oakley and Hooligan define hypnosis as a state of change in mental activity after an induction procedure that mainly includes concentration and absorption. Importantly, in the hypnotic state, the implied subjects are more likely to respond to the hypnotic recommendations, which are statements that are induced or after the purpose of changing or affecting behavior. They may include pain relief, exercise paralysis, or post-hypnotic amnesia.

Recent cognitive neuroscience studies have successfully demonstrated the impact of these recommendations on potential brain activation using objective neuroimaging methods. In terms of treatment, hypnosis has proven to be a useful tool for reducing pain, anxiety, and stress-related diseases, and several studies have provided evidence for the beneficial effects of anesthesia on sleep disorders and insomnia.

Enjoy your reading!

Guided Hypnosis to Improve Insomnia

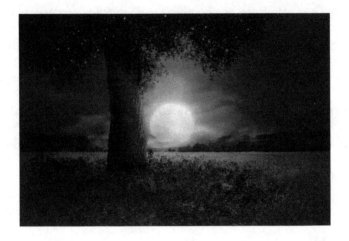

Hypnosis may remind people of the image of people rattling like ducks on stage, but the reality is that it is usually more tedious and can induce sleep. Yes, hypnosis may be a tool for people who are fighting various sleep disorders, such as insomnia or sleepwalking. For people with insomnia, hypnosis can help the body and mind relax and eliminate the anxiety of being unable to fall asleep. On the other hand, sleepwalkers can learn through hypnotic advice and wake up when his feet land on the floor. Hypnosis may also increase the time you spend in slow-wave sleep (deep sleep) by up to 80%. That is critical because deep sleep is essential for memory and recovery, so you will feel recovered when you wake up.

What is Insomnia?

Insomnia defines as difficulty falling asleep or falling asleep for a long time until you feel refreshed the next morning. Most of us will experience sleep disruption and will know how you feel when you can't seem to fall asleep. It may be that you are thinking about the next day, or drinking coffee too quickly before going to bed. Maybe you find it easy to fall asleep, but you will still wake up all night. Either way, rough sleep will make you feel exhausted and irritable the next day—those who suffer from insomnia experience these feelings regularly. It estimates that one-third of people in the UK have insomnia episodes throughout their lives. Although it can affect anyone at any age, people over 60 and women seem to be more vulnerable.

Types of Insomnia

There are many types of insomnia, but they usually divide into two categories:

Temporary Insomnia

If insomnia lasts from one night to three or four weeks, it classifies as temporary or acute. Common causes of transient insomnia include jet lag, changes in daily or working conditions, stress, caffeine, and alcohol. Some cases of temporary insomnia are called transient or intermittent insomnia. That is when the person regularly encounters sleep problems for months or years.

Persistent Insomnia

It is also known as chronic insomnia. Usually, the problem lasts for at least four weeks almost every night. Drugs that may be due to pain or medical conditions often disrupt sleep. These may include arthritis, Parkinson's disease, asthma, allergies, hormone changes, or mental health problems.

Unlike what you think, hypnosis does not occur by watching the swing of a pocket watch. That can usually be done by listening to the hypnotherapist's verbal prompts, which will put you into a like state, which can compare to indulging in excellent tips to mediate the surrounding environment. For example, a meeting designed to help you sleep deeper may use words like "relax," "deep," and "relaxed" to make a soft and soothing sound. Afterward, you may lose sleep even while listening, although some people describe hypnosis as making people feel extremely relaxed, during hypnosis, your brain focuses on deep concentration.

Hypnosis may be better for some people. That is because some people are "easier to understand" than others; that is, they are more likely to fall into a hypnotic state. However, about a quarter of people cannot hypnotize. Were you interested in trying it? People who use hypnosis to help solve sleep problems see the results in just a few meetings, so you don't have to make a big commitment. Hypnosis is not an independent treatment of sleep disorders, but another tool that can be tried, usually practiced by doctors, nurses, and psychotherapists. Talk to your doctor about referrals.

If you look up the term "insomnia" in the dictionary, you will see that it defines as unable to sleep. But this is only a small part of the story. People with insomnia often have difficulty falling asleep and staying asleep. If you have insomnia, you are likely to experience one or more of the following conditions regularly:

- You find it hard to fall asleep at night.

- You wake up at night.

- You wake up early and can't sleep.

- You get tired after getting up.

- You will feel tired during the day, irritable, and have difficulty concentrating.

- You find it difficult to take a nap during the day even if you are tired.

According to the NHS website in the UK, you may experience these problems for months or even years. It was a long time. Do you agree to a good night's sleep? Do you agree? The average adult needs 7 to 9 hours of sleep each night. But why? Why is sleep so important? Why can't you stay awake? You will do more, and you may never fall behind again, right? So why go to bed first?

Well, it turns out that if you don't get enough sleep, you may die. (Yes, this is important!) It has found that mice that do not sleep will die within 2 to 3 weeks. That's when they starved to death. Sleep not only allows you to rest, although it is part of sleep. When you sleep, your body and mind are doing amazing things.

A good night's sleep can improve learning ability. With enough sleep, you can be more focused, attentive, make better decisions, and be creative. If you do not get enough sleep, research shows that you will have difficulty solving problems, controlling emotions, and coping with changes. You will be more prone to mood swings and more likely to feel depressed. You will also find it challenging to motivate. Just one sleepless night is enough to make a person irritable and clumsy. The lack of 2 nights of sleep can make a person unable to think straight and perform their routine tasks. After five nights of sleeplessness, a person is likely to start hallucinating and seeing something that does not exist.

Causes of Insomnia

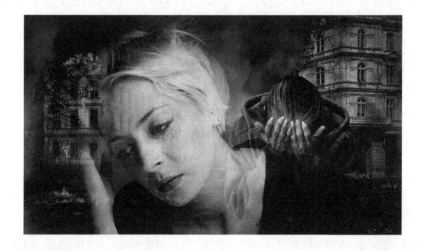

Many factors can cause insomnia. Some of these problems are easier to solve than others, such as loud noise, uncomfortable bed, drinking too much caffeine or alcohol before going to bed, or sleeping in a room that is too hot or too cold. People who work in shifts may find it difficult to fall asleep only because they feel they have the opportunity to fall asleep. Similar problems can occur with jet lag, which can also disrupt a person's typical day and night sleep patterns. These are all problems that may cause insomnia, but they are relatively small and may be transient. There are many potential causes of problems. In some cases, it may only be a cause of insomnia, while in other cases, multiple factors may encounter.

Physical Health

If you have a medical condition that causes pain, it may be difficult to fall asleep similarly, if you have a disease that affects breathing, such as asthma. It believes that hormonal problems and urinary conditions can also affect sleep patterns. The drugs you take may affect your sleep. If you suspect a health problem or think your medicine may cause your sleep problems, please consult your doctor.

Mental Health

Specific mental health problems may cause sleep problems. For example, people with severe depression are more likely to suffer from insomnia. When a person lacks sleep, the depression caused by depression also increases.

Anxiety is another disease often associated with insomnia. Stress can make people feel nervous, worried, and overwhelmed. These feelings may make it difficult to fall asleep. When trying to fall asleep, people's thinking tends to accelerate, and it feels like they can't turn off. Worries may also disrupt sleep, and the person may wake up all night. If this pattern continues, fear that lack of sleep will turn into a vicious circle.

Lifestyle

Daily habits and lifestyle influence sleep patterns. For example, if you drink regularly, you may find yourself waking up at night. Alcohol is a stimulant. Although it seems natural to fall asleep after a few drinks, it usually leads to insufficient overall sleep. Similarly, drugs and caffeine can cause sleep problems. Any drug addiction can affect your sleep style, so getting treatment is essential. If you have insomnia, it recommends reducing your caffeine intake.

Working late at night can make it difficult to turn off the brain. Shift work can cause severe damage to your internal clock and make sleep tricky. If your work (or work-related stress) causes insomnia, it may be worth reassessing your working hours. Generally, treating insomnia is useful only if you know what the root cause is. Talking to professionals such as hypnotherapists can help you discover the source of the problem.

Stress

Excessive stress can cause insomnia. If you are stressed, you may find it difficult to fall asleep. Turning off the outside world, turning off thoughts and relaxing can be difficult. Moreover, if you do fall asleep, excessive stress may mean that you have trouble falling asleep. Stress can cause tinnitus, a condition in which the brain is always on high alert. As it was unable to settle down, it seemed almost impossible to fall asleep.

When pressure is the leading cause of insomnia, medicine is simple. Get rid of stress, and you will get rid of insomnia. And, if you can't get rid of stress completely, then you need to find a way to control the pressure so that it doesn't interfere with your sleep cycle.

Irregular Sleep Time

When you go to bed, the chaotic body clock will keep you energetic. Perhaps it was because of inconsistent bedtimes, a long-haul flight from another time zone, working overnight, or changing the results of work shifts. Some people have different circadian rhythms that keep them out of sync with typical activities, so it is difficult for them to fall asleep at "normal" times.

Breathing Problems

Severe sleep may be sleep apnea, which interrupts your breathing and may wake you up hundreds of times overnight. You may not remember, but you may feel drowsy the next day. Sometimes, it is related to your weight, but not always. Nasal allergies and asthma may also interfere with your breathing. A doctor can test these conditions for you and help you manage and treat them.

Dementia

In addition to memory loss, Alzheimer's disease and other forms of dementia can also upset some people, and these are when you usually want them to fall asleep, and they will become restless. It is called "Sunset Syndrome" or "Sunset." The person may feel confused, anxious, nervous, or aggressive before falling asleep, and begin to pace, swing, or even walk away. Sometimes this behavior disappears, but sometimes it makes them sleepless all night.

Pain

Whether it is due to arthritis, chronic low back disease, fibromyalgia, cancer, or illness caused by other conditions, it may prevent you from drifting calmly or interrupting your rest. Complicating the problem is that insomnia can also cause pain to be more harmed, thus forming a cycle. You may need to treat the symptoms separately from the underlying disease.

Menopause

Usually, in middle age, the woman's body will slowly stop producing progesterone and estrogen. Hormonal changes in balance and other changes that typically occur in life at this moment will make you more sensitive to stress and other things that affect sleep. The severe hot flashes—a surge of adrenaline will raise your body temperature—may make you uncomfortable, so that you wake up sweaty, sometimes several times a night.

Anxiety

Anxiety is a feeling of worry, tension, or restlessness. Just like stress, it can involve your brain and make it difficult to relax, so you can't turn off the power and fall asleep when you need it.

You may feel anxious because of one or more of the following:

- Thinking about past events
- Worry about future events
- Feeling overwhelmed by work or other responsibilities
- Feeling nervous and unable to relax
- Feeling too much to calm yourself down

Just like stress, anxiety can make it difficult for you to fall asleep, and it can also cause you to wake up at night. That is because it is quiet at night, and your brain is less active than during the day. That makes it likely for anxious feelings to drift with the waves, destroy your thinking, and keep you awake.

Depression

People with depression may have insomnia. Frustration can make you feel that you have no energy as if you are not interested in anything. Being aggressive is a real challenge because you are fighting despair and desperate emotions. Moreover, these feelings will not disappear just because it is time to sleep. According to recent investigate, insomnia and depression "often coexist." Almost 80% of people with depression have difficulty falling asleep or fall asleep. In the past, people thought that insomnia was only a symptom of depression, but the latest idea is that insomnia is an overlapping disease that requires simultaneous treatment. From all this evidence, it is clear that the quality of life of patients with insomnia may decline.

Hypnosis and Non-hypnosis Techniques to Treat Insomnia

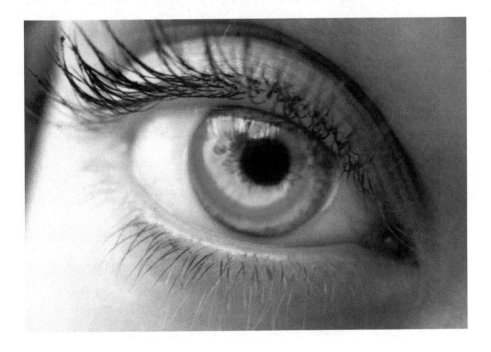

First, your subjects and clients can use many non-hypnotic strategies to solve insomnia. Therefore, before we find out how to perform hypnosis, here is a brief list of non-hypnotic methods, and provides some suggestions, you can tell them.

- Develop a sleep program—encourage your subjects to go to bed at the same time every night to establish a pattern and stick to it.

- Go to bed. And even have sex—encourage them to avoid doing other things while in bed. Reading or browsing online will put their brains at work and make it more challenging to shut down.

- Make no technical rules—the blue light emitted by the screen will inhibit the production of melatonin (sleep hormone). Therefore, either encourage them not to use them at least two hours before bedtime or download a blue light filter application to turn off blue light.

- Monitor food and beverage intake—encourage your customers to avoid caffeine consumption 4-8 hours before successful to bed. They should also attempt not to eat any food 2-4 hours before going to bed. They should go to bed and feel neither hungry nor stuffed because either feeling is enough to make them feel uncomfortable and make it hard to fall asleep.

- Do not over-exercise—they should also try not to exercise 2-4 hours before falling asleep Exercise can help people fall asleep by reducing physical stress. However, if they use too close to bedtime, they risk being overstimulated, which makes it difficult for people to open their eyes.

- Avoid drinking before going to bed—if they need to drink, encourage them to drink some water. Alcohol dehydrates the body and reduces REM sleep. That means that they are sleepier during the day and unable to concentrate.

- Practice 4-7-8 yoga-style breathing—the idea is to inhale to 4 hours, hold your breath seven times, and then exhale eight times. These numbers may not matter, but the concept of focusing on breathing can help your clients relax, relax, and eventually fall asleep.

- Sleep in a dark room—make sure their bedroom is dark. Even the red lights on the clock or radio are enough to keep people awake.

- Practice good nutrition—eating junk food that causes indigestion will prevent good sleep. Make sure food provides all the vitamins and amino acids needed for health.

Your client or subject may have tried some of these techniques, but with little success. If so, rest assured. Here are some hypnosis techniques that you can use, which can help you and your hypnosis client fall asleep and stay there.

Revival

Resurrection is a very dense memory, and your subjects can restore the mind to a certain extent. That is not the current full return they want—that know that is with you, but lost in memory and that kind of mind. It can be a great thing to regain your previous sleep experience. You can also add post-hypnotic advice so that each time your subjects perform unusual physical movements (such as touching their cheeks), they are encouraged to fall asleep. That must be unusual, they don't do it every day, because otherwise, they might fall asleep at work. Or in other daytime activities, this can be embarrassing or dangerous, or both.

Suggestions after Hypnosis

You can use it to create future memories for falling asleep. Proposals after anesthesia require two things to be effective:

- A set of instructions, when a specific event occurs, it will happen (that is, trigger)
- Results because you need triggers and results
- The bed is the right trigger.

For example: when you slip up into those sheets at night, like in other situations, you fall asleep. You have a trigger, and the trigger is the bed. Then, you let it rehearse. So, for example, if one of the belongings that prevent them from falling asleep is work-related issues, then the feeling of going to work maybe this: There is a big problem at work that you are thinking about when you go home. Perhaps you take 4-7-8 breaths to clear your thoughts. Then, you slide into bed and enter a deep sleep full of beautiful dreams.

You will practice different scenarios, in which they may not fall asleep, but will eventually fall asleep, which provides a way forward for the mind. That can be

28

accomplished through a straightforward lightning-based future memory method, in which they can mentally train to fall asleep in all these different situations.

Hypnosis Story

A great story model that can use is the "My Friend John" technique, which can use like progressive relaxation induction. My friend John (or Jane) went to bed. At first, his feet were tired, his hands were tired, his breathing became fatigued, his eyes became exhausted, and he fell asleep unconscious. By repeating this operation over and over again, you can set a pattern for them to follow. Also remember that stories can carefully design and used as a medium to deal with stress, anxiety, or other problems that cause sleep problems.

Unconscious Collection

Sleep is not something you can do consciously. The unconscious set is about learning to trust the unconscious and let the unconscious mind do things. The core of this method is to create classic, but straightforward hypnosis phenomena, such as arm suspension, and then link it to the desired hypnosis result.

E. g.: I wonder if that arm will teach you about falling asleep at night? Maybe when you sleep at night, you will feel your arms lying comfortably in bed, you will quickly drift to sleep, and your hands can only float to your knees as soon as your unconscious mind, so everything you do prepare yourself at night. Take a breath of 4-7-8, go to bed, once you feel yourself in bed and feel the temperature of your right hand, then the unconscious person can take over. The next thing you know is morning and you sleeping all night, you will feel refreshed and alert.

Sleep Phenomenon

When you fall asleep at night, you usually encounter a series of phenomena. What happens at the beginning of sleep is not encoded in memory. In other words, you don't remember the moment when you slept. The symptoms of falling asleep can suggest because it recommends that these subjects can meditate to make them fall asleep. Breathing frequency is an example. As you approach sleep, your breathing tends to slow down. Let focus on breath, rather than intentionally prolonging it, because it will generate more consciousness.

The trick is to make your hypnotic object pay attention to the moment when exhalation ends and the moment before inhalation begins. By focusing on the end of the expiration, the ideological motivation response will tend to improve the law of attention. Where attention is focused, energy flows; if you focus on the end of the expiration, the period will become longer and longer. The longer the exhalation time, the more balanced the oxygen levels in the blood, and the more likely they are to fall asleep.

Sleep Attacks 2

That is a progressive relaxation technique. The idea is to start with the feet first, and then imagine someone putting a warm blanket on their feet, slowly crossing the legs, all the way to the torso, all the way to the neck, and not reporting the unconsciousness until they touch their heads. It again depends on the "Attention Act." When you focus on the comfort zone, the comfort level will gradually increase and deepen. Is it comfortable for them to fall asleep? No, this is because they have been focusing on comfort and keeping their attention away from stressful thoughts. That allows them to do something consciously, and support is also continually developing. That may be the source of the idea of counting sheep, which puts the brain in a natural and less stressful scene and keeps it long enough to engage engaged.

Sleep Attacks 3

You will experience this. If you are addicted to an idea before falling asleep, it will become more and more vivid as you pass by. That is part of the hypnosis process, which occurs between waking and falling asleep. At that time, mental images and sounds became more vivid. The external world feels far away, so you will feel a separation from the international experience to the subjective experience. Let your theme imagine a relaxing scene, and this is the ideal place to relax. When they are addicted to the stage, it will naturally become more vivid. They don't have to try to make it more vivid, take a break until it becomes more vivid.

Another Hypnotic Phenomenon

The idea of your subject becomes disconnected. That cannot follow the same plans for logical development. It jumps from one to another, and then to another, it isn't easy to maintain the logic flow or meaning. By proposing a calm but disconnected way of thinking, two things happened:

- They can't be addicted to the thought cycle as they cause problems.

- It again reflects the phenomenon of sleep onset, hypnotic techniques listed above can use, but if you combine them into an important method, you can cook on fire! Your theme will start to believe that they can exert their power!

For example, you can let your subject follow an idea until they start jumping around the location. Let jump and be curious about where that jump to the next place. One of these ideas may elicit visual images, such as a relaxed scene or relaxed memory in nature. When this happens, they can unconsciously rest their consciousness, and then let the scene expand and consume them again and put them into the world of sleep. Pay attention to your language. For example, by saying "focus," you take the risk of making think too hard and not relax. But to say: "Let your consciousness dissipate, hover, and continue down"—this often makes the image smoother.

That is, if you find that these techniques take too long, then you can make the subjects pay attention to their breathing and be curious about the respiration and the time it takes. As time gets longer and longer, those disconnected thoughts will begin to appear, the images will start to look, comfort and relaxation will begin to spread, and somewhere in these mixes, they will fall asleep. That gives them a lot of morbidities that can happen to it.

Symptoms of Insomnia

Symptoms vary according to individual circumstances. However, there are some common symptoms, including:

- Awake for a long time at night.
- Cannot sleep, and woke up several times at night.
- Woke up very early and could not sleep.
- Feeling tired and depressed the next morning.
- I find it difficult to concentrate or work properly.
- I was feeling irritable.

Treatment of Insomnia

When treating sleep problems, you can take a variety of methods. It is essential to talk to your doctor first to eliminate any physical causes. Your doctor may recommend that you take medicine to help you fall asleep. For some people, this may be an effective treatment, but it is essential to try to find the root cause of the problem. Behavioral therapy and talk therapy are also generally recommended.

Hypnosis therapy is another treatment option that many people think is effective. Insomnia hypnotherapy can solve any potential causes while helping you relax and fall asleep. For example, if anxiety or depression is the source of your insomnia, hypnosis, and falling asleep may complement your existing treatments. Overcoming these problems may help improve your sleep style. Or, if a habit causes your insomnia (such as drinking alcohol), hypnotherapy for insomnia can break that habit.

Changing your sleep habits and solving any problems that may be related to insomnia, such as stress, medical conditions or medications can enable many people to return to a peaceful sleep. If these measures do not work, your doctor may recommend that you take cognitive behavioral therapy and medications to help improve relaxation and sleep.

Cognitive Behavior Therapy for Insomnia

Cognitive-behavioral therapy for insomnia (CBT-I) can help you control or eliminate the negative thoughts and behaviors that keep you awake. It usually recommends as the first-line treatment for patients with insomnia. Generally, CBT-1 is equivalent or more effective than sleep medication.

The cognitive part of CBT-I teaches you to recognize and change beliefs that will affect your ability to sleep. It can help you control or eliminate negative thoughts and worries that keep you awake. It may also involve removing cycles that may increase, in which you are anxious about falling asleep and not being able to fall asleep. The behavior part of CBT-I helps you develop good sleep habits and avoid behaviors that prevent you from falling asleep. Strategies include, for example:

- **Stimulation control therapy**. This method helps eliminate the factors that restrict your mind from resisting sleep. For example, you may require to train to set a consistent bedtime and wake-up time, avoid naps, only use the bed for rest and sex life, if you cannot fall asleep within 20 minutes, then leave the bedroom, only sleepy.

- **Relaxation skills**. Progressive muscle relaxation, biofeedback, and breathing exercises are ways to reduce bedtime anxiety. Practicing these techniques can help you control your breathing, heartbeat, muscle tension and mood, and relax you.

- **Sleep restriction**. This treatment reduces the time you lie in bed and avoids naps during the day, which leads to some lack of sleep, which makes you more tired the next night. Once sleep is improved, your bedtime will gradually increase.

- **Stay passive and awake**. Also known as paradoxical intent, this therapy for learning insomnia aims to reduce the anxiety and anxiety that people can fall asleep because they are lying in bed and trying to stay awake instead of falling asleep.

- **Phototherapy**. If you fall asleep too early and then wake up too early, you can use light to push back the internal clock. You can go outside when there is light out at night during the year, or you can use the lightbox.

Discuss with your doctor some recommendations or other strategies related to your lifestyle and sleep environment to help you develop habits that promote good sleep and alertness during the day.

Hypnotic Sleep

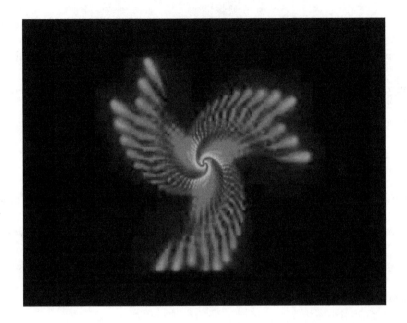

Although some sleep problems have apparent causes, others may not. If you are unsure why sleep is severe, you can use hypnosis to treat insomnia. Hypnosis therapists use a variety of techniques to discover the possible causes of problems subconsciously. Once you find the reason, you can start a tailored treatment by a hypnotherapist. During long periods of insomnia, patterns of sleep disturbances may embed in your subconscious mind. The purpose of insomnia hypnosis is to communicate with this and suggest positive changes. These suggestions will try to break down the negative thinking patterns that cause problems.

An important part of hypnosis treatment for insomnia is to teach you how to relax. For some people, physical or mental tension can make sleep difficult. Hypnosis therapists can use relaxation techniques such as progressive muscle relaxation to help reduce stress. Usually, your hypnotherapist will teach you to hypnotize yourself. That can help you develop routines and learn how to deal with triggers that cause problems. Using hypnotics to treat insomnia at home can help you bring the tools you learned in the meeting room to your daily life.

The number of hypnotic treatments you need depends on your situation. Some people only need one conversation, while others may need more in-depth work. A preliminary consultation with your hypnotherapist will give you a better understanding of how many treatments you may need.

Tips for Improving Sleep Habits

Relaxation is an essential part of effective hypnosis therapy. It is necessary to practice some self-help skills at home to enhance your experience. Improve sleep hygiene by doing the following:

- Create a routine. Try to go to bed at the same time every day.

- Exercise regularly. Exercise helps reduce stress, and exercising your body can fatigue you.

- Reduce alcohol, caffeine, and nicotine. Use herbal tea instead of tea and coffee.

- Avoid eating big meals late at night. Eat something at night. Large meals make it harder for your body to shut down during digestion.

- Relaxation is a top priority. Spend some time in the evening, taking a hot bath or reading.

- Place electronic equipment outside the bedroom. Research has found that electronic devices can affect sleep. Try to put them outside the bedroom and stop using them an hour before going to bed.

- Write a to-do list. If you are busy thinking about everything you need to do the next day, then sleep may be difficult. Eliminate trouble and write it down.

- Make your bedroom more comfortable. Make sure your bed and pillows are soft and keep the room cold and dark.

Can Hypnosis Treat Insomnia?

Hypnosis is a complementary or alternative therapy that involves deep relaxation and concentration. During hypnosis, people will be awake, but they have less understanding of their surroundings and may respond less to stimuli (including pain). Some studies have shown that hypnosis can effectively control chronic pain, reduce anxiety, and reduce anxiety, especially when combined with cognitive-behavioral therapy (CBT) and mindfulness therapy. Some studies have shown that hypnosis therapy can help treat insomnia or undesirable behavior during sleep, such as sleepwalking. Therefore, it is reasonable to assume that hypnosis can relieve patients with chronic insomnia.

The medical efficacy of mind and body therapy is an emerging scientific field, so information about the therapeutic benefits of hypnosis is limited. Research results about the effectiveness of hypnosis in insomnia are mixed. An overview of published studies on this topic shows that sleep is beneficial in 58% of the reviews. Many studies on this subject have small sample sizes or inconclusive results, so experts recommend conducting more studies to determine whether hypnosis is more effective or more effective than drugs or CBT in treating sleep disorders.

Despite the limited clinical evidence, many people report that hypnosis promotes a sense of calm, relieves anxiety and anxiety, and helps sleep. Unlike sleeping pills, hypnosis has no side effects, so it expects to be an insomnia treatment for those who do not want or want to take sleeping pills. Currently, there are no FDA approved sleeping pills for children. That means that children with insomnia must treat with other methods. Although changes in CBT and sleep hygiene can help children with sleep problems, hypnosis may be a useful treatment tool in combination with other therapies. Some people think that children are more likely to enter trance than pre-pubertal children, which makes hypnosis more active than adults. A new study found that hypnosis can effectively treat adolescents' various physical discomforts, from headaches to sleep disorders.

In other words, we have insufficient sleep for a long time, and this lack of sleep limits the body's ability to repair and recover. But insomnia, sleep hypnosis may provide solutions to help us fall asleep faster. Sleep is essential to health. During sleep, our bodies will naturally recover. Restore hormone levels, rejuvenate the spirit, and undergo various critical health processes. In short, when we lose quality sleep, we put our physical and mental health at risk. Unfortunately, resetting the biological clock to achieve a deep, peaceful sleep is not always easy.

How Can Hypnosis Help People with Insomnia?

In short, many sleep disorders burry in our subconscious mind. At bedtime, drowsiness replaces by anxiety. We let the pressure envelope our thoughts, and as a result, we seem unable to close the internal dialogue and fall asleep. However, insomnia hypnosis provides a solution. Sleep hypnosis offers a roadmap for preparing, relaxing, and inducing sleep. Hypnosis can help us overcome the restlessness of bedtime, relax our body and mind faster, and finally enter a night of deep restorative sleep.

Why is it Helpful for Insomnia?

In short, sleep, or insomnia hypnosis is a technique for inducing deep sleep, which is similar to traditional hypnosis. At bedtime, you can follow the steps to achieve physical and mental relaxation. Once you reach the state of relaxation and concentration, the system will provide you with recommendations to help your brain go to sleep.

You can try hypnosis to treat insomnia if:

- You have a hard time falling asleep.

- At bedtime, your mind moves at a rapid pace to prevent your mental breakdown.

- It is difficult for you to fall asleep before an important event occurs;

- Or you have a specific sleep disorder, such as restless leg syndrome, night terrors, or sleepwalking.

The power of good night

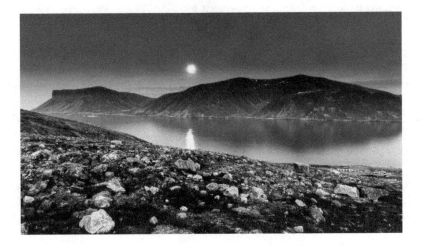

Sleep is the medicine of nature. Researchers have linked sleep deprivation to severe various health consequences. For example, adequate sleep has shown to reduce the risk of heart disease, stroke, and diabetes. But lack of sleep can also affect our quality of life. It can affect:

- Poor sleep can reduce sexual desire.

- It can accelerate the aging process.

- It affects our emotions and is the root cause of depression.

- It destroys our memories, making it more difficult to recall and store memories.

- It impairs our ability to reason, focus, and solve problems during the day.

However, you cannot just sleep more to reverse some symptoms. On the contrary, deep sleep is the most important.

At night, you will go through four sleep stages. During the NREM cycle, you will experience light sleep (N1) and sleep onset (N2), and then enter a deep restorative sleep mode (N3). Finally, you have reached the most critical REM sleep, which supports mental and physical functions, in which brain waves slow down, and the body recovers on its own. Unfortunately, in our 30s and 40s, our ability to enter deep sleep begins to weaken, and we are more likely to experience non-refreshing sleep.

Can Hypnosis Help You?

When you do not have enough slow-wave sleep, you may show many storytelling systems. If you continue to experience these symptoms, you can start a sleep hypnosis program. Common symptoms include:

- Irritability or drowsiness during the day
- Troubles keep awake
- Inattention, difficulty in concentrating, memory and attention
- Unable to control emotions
- Feeling tired at noon in the afternoon
- Slow response time

How can hypnosis help you fall asleep? Many reasons may exacerbate your sleep difficulties. For example, anxiety and stress are the two most important factors that can impair your ability to "turn off" your brain before going to bed. Diseases such as allergies or asthma can also keep you awake. Or the reason may seem to be irrelevant to regular changes.

However, in many cases, we remain sober about internal dialogue. That is how insomnia and hypnosis can help. You may think about the upcoming stress event and compete. (Like the first day of work]. Otherwise, you may replay unresolved problems from your mind over and over again. (For example, a fight with a spouse or a meeting where a dispute occurs at work). Insomnia Sleep Hypnosis provides a framework that can help us close our minds, bring our bodies to a state of relaxation, and eventually make us fall asleep from hypnosis. In particular, the hypnosis that promotes sleep can help you:

Body Relaxation: Hypnosis usually provides steps to relieve body tension, relax muscles and achieve bodyweight. Under hypnosis, the body can relax completely, which can make through breathing and focusing techniques.

Mental Relaxation: Hypnosis is like meditation, a state of increased consciousness and attention. By following the hypnotic technique, you can reduce the burden. You seek to get rid of your conscious thoughts and get out of touch with your surroundings. This type of sleep hypnosis is useful because it can help you slow down your inner thoughts, adjust your thoughts, or focus your attention elsewhere.

Causes Sleep: Contrary to popular belief, hypnosis does not sleep. You remain conscious and conscious. But the transition from trance to sleep is natural. They have similarities, so once you relax; a simple suggestion can help you fall asleep.

Falling into A Deep Sleep: Studies have shown that listening to sleep hypnosis recordings before bed can help us enter deep sleep faster. A 2014 study found that women who looked to sleep hypnosis recordings before going to bed spent 80% more on deep sleep. In other words, hypnosis can help us fall asleep faster and sleep longer, ensuring that we spend enough time in the required N3 and REM sleep stages.

Hypnosis Therapy Helps Insomnia

Insomnia is the most common sleep disorders. For chronic patients, this condition may seriously affect the quality of life. There are many types of insomnia. Insomnia can be short-term. For example, changes in routines, illness, hormones, sadness, or anxiety may make it difficult to fall asleep. Fortunately, in most cases, you will return to your regular sleep schedule within a few days or weeks.

On the other hand, chronic insomnia refers to a persistent long-term sleep disturbance. If you are unable to fall asleep for more than a few months three weeks a week, you may feel insomnia long-term. Also, insomnia can regard as "sleep onset" or "maintenance of sleep" insomnia. Sleep onset refers to difficulty falling asleep, while sleep maintenance refers to trouble falling asleep. Hypnosis can alleviate the root cause of all types of insomnia.

Long-Term Insomnia

People with chronic insomnia tend to be anxious about falling asleep; they make their minds think it will be difficult to fall asleep. This adjustment deeply burry in the subconscious mind. Through hypnosis, these people can begin to reconstruct these subconscious minds and generate more positive associations. For example, during sleep hypnosis, a recording or hypnosis therapist may use positive words such as "peace," "rest" or "rest" to describe bedtime and sleep time. That helps the subconscious to unravel its negative associations.

Acute Insomnia

For acute patients, sleep hypnosis provides a step-by-step process to regulate sober thoughts, achieve a state of physical and mental relaxation, and prepare the body and mind for bed rest. Acute insomnia usually results from stress or anxiety. You are thinking about the day, or feeling stressed about the upcoming events. By using hypnosis, you can provide a framework for your brain to shut down the system more effectively.

Hypnosis and Sleep Disorders

In addition to insomnia, deep sleep hypnosis can also help relieve a series of other sleep disorders and diseases. Studies have shown that hypnosis can effectively overcome jet lag, night terrors, and sleepwalking.

Jet Lag

Travelling can disrupt your sleep plan and may confuse your internal clock. Sleep hypnosis provides a way to reset the internal clock. For example, after returning to China, you may be hypnotized one week before going to bed. By using self-hypnosis techniques, you can encourage the body to relax at regular times and return to your schedule faster.

Restless Leg Syndrome

Restless leg syndrome refers to a state where people feel irritable. Usually, it feels out of control. However, what some people do not know is that RLS can significantly disrupt sleep. That is a common cause of insomnia because patients cannot stay still at night and will eventually toss and turn. Stress and anxiety thought to exacerbate symptoms. Hypnosis can provide a way to overcome potential causes. In particular, an asleep hypnosis treatment plan for people with RLS will provide tools to focus your mind on physical discomfort.

Dream Disease

Anyone who often experiences vivid nightmares may suffer from nightmares. Since dreams occur during REM sleep, this situation deprives individuals of the most crucial deep sleep. Fantasies may be rooted in thoughts and behavior patterns and eventually embedded in your subconscious mind—hypnosis design to re-adapt your subconscious mind to get rid of negative emotions. A hypnotic program for nightmares will seek to discover patterns, thoughts, and behaviors that may lead to repetitive dreams.

Horror at Night

Night terrors, like nightmares, can disrupt sleep throughout the night. People who suffer from night terrors are panicked and often confused or unable to communicate. Stress, sadness, and anxiety are the main factors that cause this condition. Hypnosis can help people examine the thought patterns and habits that cause night terrors.

Sleepwalking

Sleepwalking is usually portrayed as a harmless sleep disorder. The fact is: sleepwalkers are serious. It not only interferes with sleep, but also puts patients in various dangerous situations. Hypnosis therapy allows sleepwalkers to renew the subconscious mind that may cause sleepwalking. Studies have shown that clinical hypnosis is beneficial for sleepwalking. A major five-year study found that hypnosis can help two-thirds of patients eliminate or significantly reduce symptoms.

For many of these situations, it may be helpful to work with a professional hypnotherapist. Professionals can help you delve into the subconscious and determine the habits and ways of keeping these behaviors as they are.

Sleep Hypnosis: Is It Useful?

What most people with sleep disorders want to know is: Is hypnosis effective? Ok, research shows it can. Research that conduct has been demonstrated that hypnosis can have a positive effect on insomnia, RLS, nightmares and night terrors, and sleepwalking. The research on self-hypnosis is very eye-catching. Take a look:

Slumber

For example, in 2014, Swiss researchers found that recording hypnotic records of sleep can significantly improve the sleep quality of study participants. The study found that participants who were susceptible to hypnosis fell asleep longer (66% reduction in awake time), which he

lped them to enjoy deeper sleep (80% more on average).

Fall Asleep Faster

Another study looked at the effect of hypnotic relaxation four times a week on the rate at which participants fell asleep. The results: During the review, participants who received hypnotic therapy fell asleep faster than the placebo and control stimulation groups. Try to fall asleep immediately.

Night Terror

A 2007 study examined the effects of hypnosis on various sleep disorders, including sleepwalking and night terror. Participants received treatment only once, but after one month, 55% said they did not spell or have improved a lot. A similar study conducted in 1991 studied the effects of self-hypnosis on sleepwalking and night terror. Instruct patients on how to use self-hypnosis at home and require them to follow the procedure regularly. At the end of the study, 74% of patients reported feeling "significantly improved."

Various Conditions

Finally, psychology researcher Alfred Barrios examined a series of studies that compared the effectiveness of psychoanalysis and hypnosis as treatments for sleep disorders, addiction, and other diseases.

Hypnosis Quick Tips

That is good news: you can try hypnosis at home before going to bed tonight. Guided hypnosis recordings or self-hypnosis programs design to help you relax and relax, which may be the answer to sleep problems. You can use three media for hypnosis tests. You can try:

- **Sleep self-hypnosis**: Self-hypnosis refers to the steps you can take to induce the induce state, relax the body, and provide useful suggestions to the brain. Before going to bed, you should follow the sleep hypnosis script, which may include breathing techniques, mindfulness techniques, and relaxation strategies. Then, you will recite a script to help you fall asleep.

- **Guided self-induced recording**: A guided hypnosis course is an audio or video recording that features a hypnotist to provide you with relaxation techniques and strategies. Then, the hypnotist will offer some simple suggestions to help the brain go to sleep. The script may include active sleep works, such as "letting go," "yawning" or "peace," which will help you unconsciously transition from the mind state to the sleep state. A typical recording lasts about 15 minutes. Browse all our "insomnia" sleep records now.

- **One-to-one hypnosis therapy**: a meeting with a professional hypnotherapist provides personalized guidance. The hypnotist will guide you through the relaxation techniques to reach the hypnotic state, and then help you to check the subconscious and rebuild negative associations. One-to-one conversations are especially useful for entrenched sleep disorders (such as night terrors or sleepwalking) or self-hypnosis that do not provide the results you want.

No matter which method you choose, remember that hypnosis requires investment. You must first want and promise to see the results, just like any self-improvement plan. If you don't have immediate results, don't be discouraged. On average, it takes six meetings to achieve results, and some sessions may require maintenance meetings in the next few years. For self-hypnosis, long-term adherence to a program can help you achieve your goals.

The Effect of Insomnia on the Brain

Scientists and health experts have long known the critical link between quality sleep and improved mental health. Still, for many years, the root causes of insomnia that were not caused by medical disorders or the use of stimulants have troubled them. A recent study compared the sleep status of ordinary sleepers and insomniacs and examined the effect of insomnia on the brain using MRI imaging. The results showed that patients with insufficient sleep have weakened connections in the thalamus (the brain region that controls sleep and consciousness).

Although researchers cannot determine whether the weakened thalamus connection is the real cause of insomnia, or whether lack of sleep itself causes vulnerable connections, this study provides important clues to the occurrence and treatment of insomnia. Many study participants who complained of not being able to fall asleep had MRI scans, which showed that the white matter of the brain was damaged, which prove to destroy the body's biological clock and maintain the best circadian rhythm.

Researchers are not sure about the persistence of abnormal brain caused by insomnia. To be sure, lack of sleep can have a significant impact on brain and nerve function. Scientists have found that memory; attention and mood are all affected by lack of sleep and can improve sleep, concentration, and mood by improving sleep quality. Sleep experts recommend that you make regular routines during sleep to ensure that you do not cause a "sleep burden," which is a permanent lack of sleep caused by irregular sleep patterns. They recommended that everyone have at least seven hours of sleep each day, and they made it clear that the debt they catch up on when they go to bed on the weekend cannot repay.

One of the best ways to ensure adequate sleep is to focus on creating an ideal sleeping environment. You can do this by leaving the bedroom without electronics, dimming the lights, and maintaining a moderate temperature when going to bed. Your bed is also an essential part of an ideal sleeping environment. Your mattress should be comfortable and supported to promote a quality sleep- memory foam mattress found to provide the perfect combination of comfort and full-body support.

The Physiological and Psychological Effects of Insomnia

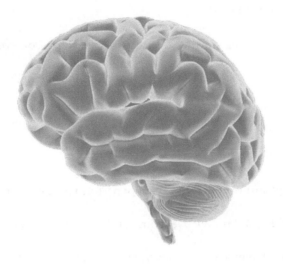

So far, we all know that sleep is an essential part of our overall health, and the fact is that rest is as indispensable as breathing or eating. When you sleep, your body will work hard, which is good for your physical and mental health and helps you prepare for the new day. Insomnia can have a severe impact on the body or even lose an hour of sleep. Every Monday night can cause energy and energy deficiency, as well as irritability and mood swings.

The long-term effects of insomnia are even more severe, leading to poor coordination and decision-making ability, as well as medical conditions such as high blood pressure, diabetes, and thyroid disease. Harvard Medical School found that if you sleep less than five hours a day, insomnia can even increase your risk of death by as much as 15%. Let's take a look at the adverse effects of insomnia on the body.

Insomnia and Your Heart

The effects of insomnia on the heart can be dangerous or even fatal. Facial cardiovascular problems with chronic lack of sleep include high blood pressure, heart disease, stroke, and high blood pressure.

Insomnia and the Brain

Insomnia can exhaust your brain and cannot perform the necessary duties to keep you happy, healthy, and productive. Some of the possible effects of insomnia on the brain include the inability to concentrate, choking creativity, short-term and long-term memory loss, and mood swings. Other risks of a sleep-deprived brain are hallucinations, mania, impulsive behavior, depression, delusions, and suicidal thoughts.

Insomnia and Stomach Pain

Weight gain is only one result of lack of sleep, and this is almost entirely due to the effect of insomnia on the digestive system. Lack of sleep can cause our body to produce too much cortical, stress hormones, and reduce the level of lepton, which is a hormone that tells us that we are full and satisfied. Insomnia also encourages the body to release higher levels of insulin, which leads to excessive fat storage and may even cause 2 diabetes.

Insomnia and Your Immune System

When we fall asleep, our bodies produce anti-infective antibodies, which help protect us from infection with viruses such as influenza and the bacteria that cause diseases such as the common cold. Insufficient sleep can weaken the immune system, which means that one of the effects of insomnia on the body is the inability to prevent and resist disease, and may even increase the risk of chronic diseases in the future.

Insomnia and Your Mental Health

The psychological effects of insomnia can also be shocking, including depression, anxiety, and even suicidal thoughts. Those who diagnosed with bipolar disorder, alcoholism, and even ADHD may find that insomnia is one of the side effects that accompany their diseases, and can also encourage their anger.

Insomnia Yoga Routine

Someone told us that we should sleep more. However, if you have insomnia, the idea of having trouble sleeping all night seems to be like dreaming. You may have tried counting the flocks before and after, so the next step may be to add gentle yoga exercises to your routine every night. Harvard Medical School's "Trusted Sources" study found that regular yoga exercises can improve sleep efficiency, total sleep time, and the rate at which participants fall asleep, as well as other improvements for patients with insomnia. Although you may feel that you should be tired after strenuous exercise before bed, you want to calm down the nervous system and relax from the day. Yoga, the key to yoga, is to maintain a calm and restorative posture. Follow this routine to get started.

Fold Forward

Forward folding is a gentle reversal, and it activates your parasympathetic nervous system. This system will slow down the body's progress. It will release stress and help you fall asleep.

- Start to stand upright with your feet separated from your hips.
- When you raise your arms and straighten out, please take a deep breath until they touch the top of your head.
- When exhaling, contract the front of the thigh to pull the knee up and bend forward from the waist.
- Inhale gently and grasp the opposite elbow, straighten it out, and hang your arms under the top of your head to stretch your body posture—if you are anxious about the balance here, and you can expand your posture.
- Before standing up slowly, take 10 to 15 deep breaths slowly.

Supine Torsion

In general, twisting helps to detoxify, release tension, and relieve back pain. Also, some reclining positions found to help relax bar reflex and lower blood pressure.

- You are lying on the mat. When inhaling, extend your knee into your chest.

- When exhaling, extend your arms to the shoulder-high side, let your knees fall to the side, and put your knees on top. If necessary, a small cushion (such as a pillow) can be placed under the lower knee to support the torque.

- When breathing, check your body to ensure that no shoulder bones lift off the ground. If so, you can raise your legs slightly and add a cushion (or another cushion) to keep your shoulders pressed into the pillow.

- Stay here and take a deep breath at least five times. When inhaling, lift your legs back to the chest, press it into your arm to help it move, and then put it on the other side.

Puppy Pose

Puppy pose is a modified child pose, and it stretches the upper back, spine, and shoulders. That helps relieve tension and stress. The forehead on the ground also stimulates the pituitary gland, which is the primary source of melatonin. Melatonin can help you fall asleep.

- Stretched muscles: *latissimus dorsi*, significant deformity, rotator cuff muscles, abdomen, deltoid into the limbs of the mat, the hips stack on the knees, and the shoulders stack on the wrists.

- Don't move your hips and start to stretch your hands forward, but don't put your elbows on the floor.

- When exhaling, tuck your toes underneath and move your hips to about half of your heels, then gently place your forehead on the cushion.

- Breathe here, keep a slight bend in your lower back, and press your hand down and stretch to your arms and spine.

- Stay here for 5 to 10 breaths, and then walk backward so that you will be okay again.

Children's Posture

Children can stretch their hips, thighs, and ankles. It can also passively stretch the back torso and gently relax the muscles of the front body. This posture can reduce stress, stimulate melatonin, and calm the mind. Stretched muscles: latissimus dorsi, lower back, shoulders, and buttocks.

- Starting from the limbs, put your big toes together, so they touch each other, widen your knees to at least the width of your hips, and then put them back on your heels.

- When exhaling, place the torso between the thighs. If you feel more comfortable, you can widen your feet or place a small long cushion between your legs to support your body.

- When you are entirely lying in the "child pose," you can extend your arms in front of you and stretch, but as a follow-up step in the "puppy pose," you can put your hands next to the torso and palms up.

- Breathe at least ten times here. When you rise from it, do so while inhaling and support you with your hands as needed.

Posture with Legs Up

The upper wall of the leg is a gentle inversion. It is also completely passive, so it can help your brain and body fall asleep.

- Move the cushion to the wall area where there is space and place it in parallel.

- Lie down with your feet on the ground and your knees bent.

- Leaning on your lower back, lift your feet and gently swing your torso so that it is perpendicular to the wall. Place the ischium on the bottom of the wall and your legs on the wall.

Overcome Insomnia and Improve Sleep

Now that you know how insomnia affects the body and mind, it's time to discuss how to beat insomnia and get the best sleep in life—no more excuses! There are many ways to embrace rest to relieve insomnia, including how to know when and how to make a new bed, drink a cup of herbal tea in the evening, or practice meditation in bed at night.

- Set a sleep schedule: going to bed and waking up at about the same time every day will help your body and mind enter an ideal sleep-wake cycle. With the set sleep schedule, you will be able to fall asleep faster, wake up brighter, and rejuvenate—we mean the same on weekends!
- Fall asleep as soon as possible: If you find yourself having to get up several times later than usual, try to make up for the lost sleep as quickly as possible, and then turn in the next night instead of falling asleep. Later, this may cause a vicious cycle, making it impossible to fall asleep the next night of the week.

- Say no to Joe: Every one of us likes to drink a good cup of coffee in the morning, but if you want to get a good night's sleep, the best option is to avoid any caffeine after 2:00 pm, because caffeinated substances can Stay in your system for six hours, so when you should prepare for sleepy time, it will excite you.

- Passing Booze at bedtime: Yes, alcohol can calm down and help you beat but sleep more quickly, but it can also cause sleep disturbances at night and prevent you from achieving the deep restorative sleep you need to be happy and healthy.

- Go to the gym in the evening: Exercise is an excellent way to increase physical strength during the day, but it often makes your core temperature increase. The body is difficult to cool, so it feels relaxed and sleepy. For best sleep, avoid strenuous exercise at least three hours before going to bed.

- Cooling down: Sleep experts have found that the ideal sleeping temperature is between 60°F and 68°F. That is because the body needs to stay calm to fully relax, but not too cold to adapt to natural protection needs. Its core temperature starts from immersion too low. Keeping the bedroom at about 65 degrees Fahrenheit at night should be the best place to go to the Dreamland.

- Keep a low profile: You also want to keep dim lights in your bedroom to encourage the production of melatonin, a sleep hormone that plays a vital role in helping you get quality sleep every night. It would help if you also avoided bright lights a few hours before going to bed.

- Abandon your equipment: put the electronic equipment outside and make your bedroom a safe haven! The best option is to completely exclude everything that emits "blue light"—this means no TV, iPod, Smartphone, etc. However, if you have to put the electronic device in the bedroom, make sure to turn it off at least two hours before going to bed to avoid any irritating effect on them.

- Take some time to relax: every night you can do some of the most important things to promote a better sleep, which is to set aside half an hour to relax before going to bed. Your body needs a buffer between the stress of the day and the rest of the night. You can help your body get, thereby participating in your favorite relaxation activities. You can drink a cup of warm herbal tea, read a book, take a hot bath, or even practice some simple yoga moves.

- Invest in a better bed: If you have tried all the methods but still seem to be unable to meet the other functions you need, then you may need to consider investing in a premium memory foam mattress and then bid farewell to a block-shaped built-in spring bed. Memory foam proves to provide therapeutic spinal support, reduce joint pressure through even weight distribution, and provide a cooling effect for the ideal sleep temperature.

Buddhist Meditations

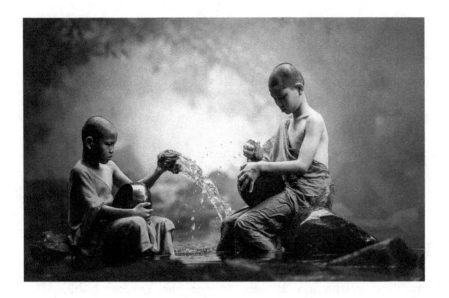

Mindfulness Meditation

The practitioners of mindfulness meditation focus on the present moment, accepting and not appreciating any thoughts, emotions, sensations. If the mind is distracted and begins to wander, at the moment of awareness, it is necessary to return it to breathing or observing the present moment. The practice of mindfulness consists not only in meditation while sitting or lying down, but also during daily activities: eating, walking, in transport, or at work. The meditation of awareness in everyday life is to pay attention to the present moment, to be aware of what is happening right now, and not to live in an automatic mode.

If you are speaking, you need to pay attention to the words, how you pronounce them and listen with care. If you are walking, pay attention to the sensations in the body, sounds, smells, and people around you. The daily practice of mindfulness helps to meditate while sitting, and vice versa.

Who is Mindfulness Meditation for?

This type of meditation is suitable for the general public. It is recommended that you begin to meditate with it. It is used in schools, hospitals, and other institutions to help people reduce their exposure to stress, improve their physical and psychological health, and improve their living standards.

Awareness meditation does not affect aspects of Buddhist philosophy, rituals, etc. Therefore, it is suitable for people who want to get only the benefits of meditation to improve their health. If you are interested in a more in-depth spiritual development, then meditation of awareness can be your first step toward this goal.

Zen Meditation (Sitting Meditation)

Sitting meditation is one of the Buddhist practices aimed at realizing one's true nature, conducted in a sitting position with legs crossed (or in a lotus position), with a straight back and hands folded in front of you.

In Japan, zazen is often perceived merely as one of the spiritual practices, without connecting it only with any particular religion or Buddhist school. Ordinary people can practice zazen under the guidance of Buddhist monks in temples. In cities, many churches provide an opportunity to familiarize themselves with this practice. It is done either for free or for a small fee, usually up to 1,500 yen. Often the size of the cost is not set, and in such cases, the participant decides whether to pay or not, and if he chooses to pay, the amount is determined by himself.

Monk Staff Helps Meditation

One of the unusual features of zazen for meditation is the use of the kayaks stick, as called in the Rinzai school (in Zen Buddhism, Soto - Kiyosaki). During meditation, a person loses focus, posture changes, and is overcome by drowsiness - in such cases, a monk who watches meditation hits a person on the shoulder with a stick. The purpose of this is to draw attention to the error, and the sounds of beats in the silence of the meditation hall are quite impressive. Of course, they beat not very painfully and without causing injuries.

The essence of zazen is to comprehend your nature and get rid of delusions, realizing the void core of being. Practitioners sit without thoughts, moving away from the all-consuming bustle of everyday life. The pacifying practice of zazen is accessible to everyone.

How to Practice Zen Meditation?

Meditation can be an invaluable stress reliever. If you experience stress and anxiety for one reason or another, experiment with different meditation techniques. Zen´s meditation includes a concentration on the breath and the present. First, find a convenient place and a comfortable position for yourself. Start with short breathing sessions. Over time, develop a suitable model for yourself. At first, meditation can be difficult, since the ability to free the mind comes with practice, but in the end, you will find an algorithm that will have a positive effect on you.

Method 1: Take the Right Position

1. **Create a peaceful environment where you can sit**: It is important to meditate in a friendly place without distractions. Find a relatively quiet place in your home and take steps to create a relaxing environment. It largely depends on your personal preferences. Some people like to create an altar using items such as shells, stones, or flowers. Others wish to light candles. Pick items that appease you to arrange a suitable place for meditation. Over time, your site will evolve naturally, so don't worry if it doesn't turn out perfect right away. When you begin to meditate regularly, you will understand what suits you and what does not.

2. **Take a steady position:** The literal translation of zazen is "sedentary meditation." How you sit is very important. And the most important thing is to continue to feel comfortable and keep your back straight. If you need to, for example, cross your legs or

71

use pillows to support your back, do it. If you are flexible enough, try to take the pose of half a Lotus ("Hankafuza") or a full("Kekkafuza"). To make the pose of half the Lotus, place the left foot on the right thigh, and the right - bend under the left leg. For a full Lotus pose, place each foot on the opposite thigh. However, if both postures cause you pain, do not use them, as this may distract you.

3. **Position your head in a comfortable position**: The head position is essential for Zen meditation since it is imperative not to do anything that strains the body. Keep your head in a position that seems natural to you and does not strain your neck. Ideally, the spine should be on a par with the collar. Imagine a straight line running up the spine. Move your neck so that this imaginary line continues to cross it. Besides, it can be useful to tighten the chin to align the spine and neck.

4. **Relax your jaw and face muscles:**. Before you start meditating, pause for a moment, and feel whether the muscles of the face are tightening and jaw. You may not notice tension in this area until you pay special attention to it. Try to relax your jaw and facial

muscles as a whole before starting your meditation. If your jaw is too tight, massage your face lightly with your fingers to relax your muscles.

Method 2: Learn the Basics

1. **Breathe through your nose**: In Zen meditation, the main concentration is on the breath. It is important to breathe through the nose. Inhalation and exhalation through the nose create a cooling and warming sensation. It will make it easier for you to follow the rhythm of your breathing during meditation.

2. **Concentrate on breathing**: When you begin to meditate, watch your breath as much as possible. Pay attention to the natural rhythm of inspirations and expirations, breathing, and the warm and cold sensations created by the air passing through the lungs. Try to concentrate as much as possible on your breath during the meditation session. Perhaps, at first glance, this task will seem simple to you, but it's not so simple to calm the mind. Do not give up, if at first, it will be difficult for you to concentrate on breathing. Meditation, like everything else, requires practice.

3. **Decide what to do with the eyes**: You can keep them open, half, or completely closed. It helps some people to focus on one point in the room. Others prefer to close their eyes. It is a matter of personal preference. Decide what to do with your eyes, based on what seems to you the most natural and peaceful. All this will come by trial and error. Change your mind about your eyes if you are distracted or uncomfortable. For example, if your eyes begin to watery when you focus on one point in the room, close them. Check if this helps you focus better on breathing.

4. **Redirect the mind when it wanders**: In silence, the brain can naturally begin to wander. When you first start meditating, you will probably find yourself thinking about other things. Most likely, you will start to think about the things you need to do or what happened earlier that day. Feeling that this is happening, calmly, without tension, redirect your thoughts to your breath. Please tune in to the natural ebbs and flows of breathing and the sensations that they create. Sometimes it helps to count breaths to regain concentration.

5. **Start with a two-minute meditation**: Zen´s meditation takes some effort. If you try to meditate too long at an early stage, you will probably find that you cannot concentrate on breathing. Start with just two

minutes of meditation at a time. As soon as it becomes more comfortable for you to meditate, you can increase this time.

Method 3: Gradually set the Mode

1. **Get a zafu or a small pillow. Zafu is a pillow specially designed for Zen meditation:** If you think Zen meditation is right for you, you can buy zafu on the Internet. With it, it will be easier for you to maintain the correct position each time you meditate.

2. **Do not worry about immediate excellence**: Beginners sometimes fear that they meditate poorly. It may be difficult for you to clear your mind and focus on breathing. Do not be discouraged and do not blame yourself. It is normal if, at first, meditation seems like a difficult task. Do not judge yourself severely and continue to exercise. Ultimately, meditation will become easier. Keep in mind that even people who regularly never meditate completely clear their minds. It is normal to stop from time to time and redirect your thoughts to your breath. Do not think that if you are distracted, then you meditate incorrectly.

3. **Increase your session time over time:** Start with short sessions and gradually lengthen them. After you feel comfortable meditating for two minutes, start adding a few more minutes each week. As a result, you can meditate longer. There is no single rule for meditation. You may find

relaxing, very long meditations (25 minutes per session) relaxing. But short sessions of 5-10 minutes may be enough. Experiment with different time frames until you find one that suits you.

Vipassana Meditation

Vipassana meditation was discovered by Buddha about 2500 years ago. By performing Vipassana meditation, the number of spiritual injuries will grow. And finally, you will be able to understand pure consciousness.

So what does Vipassana Meditation mean? To know it, you can understand it by first disassembling this word. If you divide Vipassana into Vi +Passana, "Vi" means "another viewpoint." "Passana" means "as is." Therefore, it means seeing what is as it is, from another perspective.

There is another perspective on what we feel as it is. Another way to look at it is to read the reality as it is—the power to confirm this change of fact as it is called Chie. The wisdom referred to here is different from the knowledge generally used.

We usually contact a lot of information, people and things. Contact with them has a significant impact on our hearts every day. For example, when you encounter information, people, or things that you feel are favorable, your mind changes. Conversely, when you meet information, people, or something that you feel unpleasant, your mind also changes.

In this way, contact with the outside world causes the mind to change repeatedly. The change in the heart will shake the soul. When our hearts bounced, a lot of dirt that has accumulated in our hearts since we were born is emerging in our hearts as bubbles appear on the surface of the water. It is greed, anger, anxiety, and doubt. This dirt causes people to suffer.

Vipassana meditation now keeps us from being touched by external contact by continuing to observe the real-world changes of this moment. Furthermore, it is possible to prevent and eliminate anger and greed that arise from memories and thoughts of the past that are already in my mind. Moreover, it is possible to avoid and reduce anger and greed that arise from memories and thoughts of the past that are already in my mind.

In this way, the impurities that have accumulated in my heart will purify more and more. In the end, you will be able to see pure consciousness without any imperfection. With pure consciousness, there is no more anger or greed. You will be able to follow the right path, live your life without shaking, and live a more active life.

Vipassana and Meditation

It's not called Vipassana meditation, as it is officially meaning only Vipassana. However, the term Vipassana meditation used to make it easier for the general public to understand. In the first place, meditation means "to look inside." The word Vipassana already has this meditation implication.

Therefore, meditation is not just about sitting on a cross, closing your eyes, and staying still. Meditation is something you can always do, and advanced practitioners of Vipassana meditation are always doing Vipassana meditation. Conversely, without constant Vipassana meditation, the purification of the mind is insignificant. That's because there are so many things in the world that make your heart dirty.

For example, we are always picking up trash. That's not trash pickup to clean the room, but trash pickup to store it in the room. We are willing to collect garbage and store it in our hearts. Vipassana meditation throws away all the debris that has accumulated in your heart and cleans it cleanly. A clean heart brings peace, as a cleanroom is refreshing.

Vipassana Meditation and Mindfulness

Recently, mindfulness has become popular in Europe and America. Mindfulness has been renamed as part of the Vipassana Meditation and will widely publicize. But it's something similar. Well-known companies such as Apple Computer, Microsoft, and Google are actively adopting mindfulness to calm their employees.

Why is Vipassana Meditation not Widespread?

This Vipassana meditation that can cleanse the mind was discovered in Buddha and spread around the world. Even in traditional Buddhist countries, quite a few people are practicing Vipassana meditation correctly. Also, practice is essential to the proper understanding of Vipassana meditation, and it can be difficult for some people to understand. Therefore, if the leader's guidance is not well-received at the meditation meeting, etc., the understanding of the participants may no t reach.

Besides, meditations that increase concentration (such as Samata meditations) are more popular than Vipassana meditations that eliminate mental dirt. You may be able to increase your productivity or have a mysterious experience by increasing your concentration, but you will not get rid of your spiritual stains. For example, if you use a broom to dust a room of dust, you will not be able to clean the room unless you remove it with soil. Even if the center of the room is clean, dust will collect in the corners of the room, and one day the soil will be scattered in the wind and scattered all over the place.

In a similarly focused meditation, the surface of the mind looks beautiful at first glance, but the dirt is just driving to the corners and not disappearing. Looking at the current world, we think that what we need today is Vipassana meditation that eliminates the spiritual stains. We hope that the correct transmission of Vipassana meditation will bring peace to people around the world.

For Whom is Vipassana Meditation Suitable?

Vipassana meditation is one of the most common types of meditation in the world. It is great for beginners. You can take a 10-day training course for free, if you wish, leaving a donation. Vipassana is not accompanied by ritual.

Lovely good Meditation (Metta Meditation)

Metta means kindness, benevolence, mercy. This practice also applies to Buddhist techniques. With regular exercise, meditation of loving-kindness allows you to develop empathy, empathize with other people. It contributes to the emergence of positive emotions through compassion, form a kinder attitude towards your personality, understands yourself and your path, make your life more whole. Metta meditation takes place with closed eyes in any position convenient for you. It is necessary to create feelings of love and goodwill in your heart and mind and direct them first at yourself. And then gradually at other people and living beings: relatives, friends, acquaintances, people that you dislike and frankly dislike, at all people and living beings on the planet, for the whole universe.

I wish them love, peace, kindness, the fulfillment of desires, prosperity, harmony, health, mercy, all the best and best. The more you develop a feeling of love and compassion for all living beings in the world, the more joy and happiness you can experience.

Who is Metta Meditation for?

If you answered at least one of the following statements positively, then meditation of loving-kindness will help you.

Sometimes I am strict and harsh (even cruel) with myself and others. I often get angry and resentful of people. I feel that I have problems with relationships with people. Metta meditation is especially for selfish people; it helps them become happier, get rid of stress and depression, to cope with insomnia, nightmares, anger, and aggression.

Indian Meditations

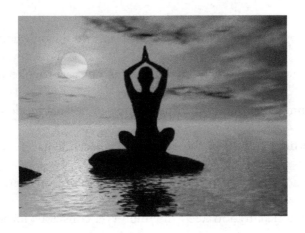

Transcendental Meditation

Transcendental Meditation (TM for short) is a technique of meditation, using mantras, founded by Maharishi Mahesh Yogi and distributed by organizations of the Maharishi Movement. In the 1970s, Maharishi became known as the guru of many stars, including the Beatles.

TM is widely practiced worldwide and has more than five million followers. There are numerous scientific studies funded by this organization that confirm the benefits of this type of meditation. Experiments confirm that TM relieves stress well and promotes personality development. However, the Maharishi Movement has critics who accuse it of sectarianism and question the authenticity of the research.

TMS is engaged in any comfortable position, and the only condition is that the head should not touch anything so as not to provoke falling asleep. The recommended duration of meditation in normal mode is 20 minutes in the morning and 20 in the evening. Transcendental meditation is not contemplation or concentration. The process of consideration and the process of concentration keep the mind at a conscious level of thinking. At the same time, Transcendental Meditation systematically transfers the mind to the source of thought, the pure field of the creative mind.

The TM technique describes as a unique and effortless process of shifting attention to more refined states of thought until the thought transcends, and the mind experiences a pure consciousness.

For whom is Transcendental Meditation Suitable?

TM course is paid and consists of seven steps: an introductory lecture, preparatory lecture, individual interview, individual training, and three days of practice. Suitable for those people who are willing to pay a certain amount of money to a licensed instructor and get a ready-made tool - TM equipment in a short time.

Advantages of Transcendental Meditation (TM Meditation)

1. Adjusting the intelligence of the body

The stresses that limit our lives result from experiencing excessive pressure and producing structural or functional abnormalities in the nervous system. The nasty reaction we have developed consists of these stresses accumulated in the body. Determining and removing stress one at a time is virtually impossible, even if we knew how to do it — although we didn't.

Fortunately, the intelligence of the body can do it. Scientifically speaking, this intelligence consists of a myriad of homeostatic feedback loops connected to blood pressure, body temperature, blood Ph, insulin levels, tissue damage, hormone levels, and many other body elements. It detects and corrects unbalances.

The stresses of our lives' enjoyment result from excessive pressures that result in structural or functional abnormalities in the nervous system.

When an imbalance is detected, the body's self-healing mechanism automatically and unconsciously balances the body's tissues and restores ideal homeostasis and health. When we get sick, our doctor may give you other instructions, but the most important thing to tell us is "take more rest." Resting makes these self-healing mechanisms work more efficiently.

2. Peaceful acuity helps relieve stress

By practicing TM, we add (but not replace) a cycle of restful agility to the normal cycle of awakening, dreams, and sleep. Restful alertness is a physiological condition that differs from these three conditions and complements the healing power. Due to its unique neurophysiological characteristics, a state of alertness full of peace is said to be one of the elements that compose the fourth state of consciousness, transcendental consciousness. The increased synchronization of EEG observed during TM practice is a manifestation of the high degree of connectivity and coordination between cortical regions of the brain, which may facilitate the body's self-healing process.

Health promotion statistics have demonstrated this health-promoting effect. A five-year study of 2,000 TM practitioners showed low subject admission rates in all disease categories, averaging 50% less. Also, subjects hospitalized 30% fewer times, demonstrating that the TMS practice of accelerating the normal healing process.

Meditation Mantra

"Man" means "mind," and "tra" means "liberate." A mantra is what frees the mind. Typically, a mantra is a syllable, word, or sentence used in meditation to focus the mind and achieve a particular emotional state.

Some people think that a mantra is a kind of affirmation and is pronounced to convince oneself of something or create an appropriate mood. It is not entirely true. Yes, each mantra has its meaning, and the vibration of sound when it is pronounced has a specific effect, depending on the value of the mantra. But the mantra is something more; it is a sacred verbal formula charged with a lot of energy and information. It can influence the consciousness of a person and help him in spiritual perfection.

The technique of performing mantra meditation is simple. It is necessary to take any of the poses for meditation, close your eyes, and repeat to yourself the chosen mantra. Sometimes practice is also supplemented by observing breathing or working with the rosary. You can meditate a certain amount of time or repetitions (traditionally 108 or 1008).

Here are some of the most famous mantras:

Om (also pronounced as AUM): For the feeling of oneness with the Lord, A - means the Personality of Godhead, U - means the Inner Energy of God, M - means living beings (like the Energy of God), and AUM - the sound vibration of the Supreme Personality of Godhead, the unity of All That Is!

Om Mani Padme Hum: Is the mantra of the goddess Guang-Yin, the goddess of mercy and compassion. The mantra is universal. It is a compelling, cleansing mantra. Plus, her practice bestows success in all areas. Mantra has a calming effect on the nervous system and helps eliminate nervous diseases.

Om Namah Shivaya: It is believed that in the five syllables of this mantra, the whole Universe is composed of five primary elements, which correlate with the chakras from Muladhara. The repetition of the mantra purifies the factors, which contribute to the internal transformation. It is Shiva who, in specific cycles of the evolution of the Universe, destroys the old world and creates a new one.

Who is the Mantra Meditation for?

Many people believe that a mantra helps them focus better and free their minds than, for example, concentration on breathing. Mantra meditation can be performed in everyday life by reciting the mantra to oneself. Some people are also attracted by the additional sacred meaning of the mantra, which gives a particular effect when practicing meditation.

Relationship Between Meditation and Mantra

One of the basic meditation methods is "close your eyes and repeat the mantra."

Meditation is the creation of a state of "thinking nothing." By emptying your head, you can rest your head and heart, which are usually stressed by stress. It's also practiced in religion, but it is not something that can do without guidance, anyone can practice it.

Sing the mantra so that it sounds to you. By chanting the mantra, it becomes easier to find the thoughts (discretion) that come to mind during meditation. If you find that you have thoughts, stop thinking, "Let's think after meditation," and return to the mantra.

In this way, we will put away the thoughts one by one. Breathing is essential when chanting the mantra.

Do abdominal breathing or Tanda breathing. Abdominal breathing. Abdominal breathing is a method of breathing in your stomach, not your chest. You can inflate your stomach by holding your ribs with both hands and inhaling. The trick is to feel the movement of the diaphragm. Tanda breathing is a breathing method that involves abdominal breathing with a strong focus on Tanda. The point is to breathe using the lower half of your tummy, not your whole stomach. Tanda is a place about 9 cm below the navel. Hold your palm from the groove to the navel with both hands and exhale slowly, practicing breathing into your tummy and get the hang of it.

Meditation Method using the Mantra

Put cushions and cushions in a quiet and calm place and cross out. It can use in either a half-waist or a half-waist.

Slowly tilt your upper body forward, put your palm on the floor, and close your eyes.

After declaring in your mind that you will enter into meditation, slowly get up for 15 to 20 seconds.

Place your left and right hands on your knees and make a circle by aligning your thumb and forefinger tips.

If you lose chest and breathe, move to abdominal breathing. While abdominal breathing or Tanda breathing, shake your upper body slightly forward, backward, leftward, and rightward to find a straight position. Repeat the mantra and enter meditation.

The thoughts that come to mind create a state of no-thought by thinking after meditation.

If you feel it's been about 15 minutes, cut off your meditation, close your eyes, and push your upper body forward.

Open your eyes when your general feeling comes back.

91

Yogic Meditations

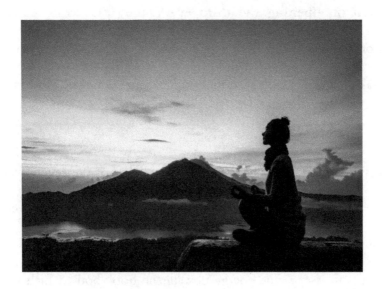

There are many types of yogic meditations. Yoga means "union." The union of body, soul, and mind. Yoga traditions are rooted very deeply in 1700 BC. And consider spiritual purification and self-knowledge to be their highest goal. Classical yoga consists of 8 components: norms and rules of behavior (Yama and Niyama), asanas (physical exercises), breathing exercises (pranayama), and contemplative meditation practices (pratyahara, Dharana, dhyana, samadhi).

Here are the most common types of yoga meditation:

Meditation on opening the third eye: During practice, attention is focused on the location between the eyebrows, called the "third eye" or "Ajna chakra." With the distraction, it must again be mentally returned to this place. The purpose of such meditation is to calm the mind.

Chakra meditation: It is necessary to choose one of the seven chakras (human energy centers) and focus on it during practice. To see its color, shape, think about its meaning, and manifest itself in your life. This meditation is to restore the energy flow in the hook body, which entails improving the quality of life in general.

Trataka meditation: It is fixing a look at an external object, such as a candle, image, or symbol (yantra). First, meditation occurs with open eyes, and then with closed eyes to train skills and concentration, and visualization. After closing the eyes, you need to restore the image of the object with your mind's eye as accurately as possible.

Kundalini Meditation: It is a comprehensive meditation practice that awakens the energy of the kundalini, which is dormant at the base of the spine. This type of meditation is recommended to be practiced only under the guidance of a qualified teacher of kundalini yoga.

Kriya Yoga: It is a set of physical, respiratory, and meditative exercises taught by Paramahamsa Yogananda. They will suit those people who are more interested in the spiritual aspects of meditation.

Nada Yoga: It is a spiritual practice based on concentration on sounds. The word "Nada" also means sound and flowering. Novice practitioners meditate on external sounds to calm the mind. Over time, they switch to the internal sounds of the body and mind. The primary purpose of such meditation is to hear the subtle vibrations of an unmanifest sound, similar to the om's sound.

Tantric meditation: In contrast to popular belief, most tantric practices have nothing to do with sexual rituals. Tantra has a rich tradition and has dozens of different meditative techniques, and quite advanced, requiring a certain degree of the calm of the mind and control of consciousness.

Who is Yoga Meditation Suitable for?

Given the wide variety of yogic meditation practices, everyone can find a meditation technique right. Meditation yoga not only resets your thoughts but also has various effects on your mind and body.

Do you Need Preparation to Start Meditation Yoga?

You don't need any special tools to start meditation yoga, but it's easier to get good results if you have an environment where you can focus on your consciousness. When beginning meditation yoga, be aware of the following:

If you have as a television or a smartphone, turn off the power to the device to be of sound aroma and incense, burn like candles, wear the right clothes comfortable to wear that does not tighten the body.

Typical Poses of Meditation Yoga

An ideal posture when performing meditation yoga is the "Lotus position." It is a pose that requires flexibility in your knees, hips, and ankles, so do it within a comfortable range.

"Lotus Position" that has the Effect of Resting and Relaxing the Brain

The pose called "Rengeza" because it looks like a lotus flower is a power charge when you put your hands on your knees, a power charge when you point your palms up, and relax when you point down. It is said to be effective. Also, set the ratio of inhaled breath to exhaled breath to 1:2 and count at a comfortable speed. Being aware of the flow of breathing will also help you to concentrate.

How to pose?

1. Sit with both legs extended forward.

2. Put your right leg firmly on your left thigh with both hands, just like crossing your legs 3. Put your left leg on your right thigh with both hands.

3. Stretch your neck and back straight as if the top of your head pulled from the ceiling.

4. Put your hands on your knees.

5. Make sure your head, neck and back are aligned.

6. Close your eyes the power of the whole body.

Points to Note When Performing Lotus Position

When performing lotus seating, it is ideal to have both knees on the floor, but if it is difficult, place a cushion or cushion under the knee to help stabilize. At first glance, the lotus position looks like sitting cross-legged, but it is a pose that requires flexibility, so please refrain from having knees or ankles with pain or malfunction.

If it is difficult to assemble the lotus position, use the "half-lotus position pose" with one leg on your thigh. It is important not to overdo it because painful postures and pain interfere with meditation.

Meditation Yoga with a Deep Sense of Liberation

Meditation is gaining increasing interest as it has introduced as part of a global corporate training program. By paying attention to your thoughts and focusing on your consciousness, you can easily notice that you are driving yourself unconsciously, and you can be free from unnecessary beliefs.

Why not give it a try if you are stressed or tend to have negative thoughts.

100

Chinese Meditations

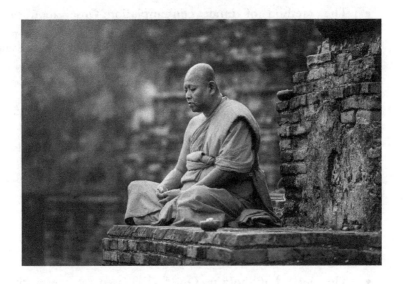

Dao Russian Meditations

Taoism is the traditional Chinese doctrine of the "way of things," which includes philosophy and religion. This type of meditation's main feature is to work with internal energy: its generation, transformation, and circulation.

The purpose of Taoist meditation aims to calm the mind and body, achieve emotional balance, and improve the circulation of internal energy and unity with Tao. Some styles of Taoist meditation are aimed at improving health and gaining longevity.

Currently practiced twelve types of Taoist meditation:

- **The method of inner contemplation:** Observation of your thoughts, feelings, emotions to calm the mind stops the endless stream of thought.

- **Center concentration method:** First, there is a distraction from the outside world, until the mind ceases to notice external sounds, visual images, and events. When the mind is calm, they move to the center - concentrating on the navel or solar plexus level to achieve equilibrium - Tao.

- **The method of "holding One.":** The essence of this meditation is to overcome division in the "I" and the outside world, to achieve integrity.

- **A method of stopping thoughts and emptying the mind:** The meaning of this meditation is to turn off the mind, without resorting to mantras entirely, or visualization, or even contemplation, to cut off all thoughts, images, feelings.

- **The method of returning to the right mind:** The purpose of this meditation is to free oneself from analytic thinking, from idle internal chatter, and develop the Tao mind, achieve a different kind of peace.

- **The method of concentration on the cavities:** The essence of this meditation is to divert attention from the outside world and concentrate on some cavity of the body to calm emotions, stop the flow of incoherent thoughts, and minimize sensations. At advanced stages, directing internal energy to a specific area of the body is practiced to clean the necessary section of the energy channel and collect energy with a view to its further purification and transformation.

- **The method of visualization of the spirit of Lozhbina:** With this meditation, the practitioner presents a specific image, and then slowly merges with it.

- **A way of emptying the mind and filling the stomach:** To empty the mind means to weaken the fire of desire, and to fill the stomach means to fill the abdominal cavity with energy. Usually, this form of meditation is practiced in combination with other techniques under the guidance of an experienced mentor.

- **A method of combining thought and breathing:** The purpose of this meditation technique is to switch from normal respiration to Tao breathing when a practitioner breathes through the nose. Still, his whole body turns into a single breath, the state of consciousness changes.

- **The method of collecting and circulating spiritual light. The technique of drawing light in.**

- **The process of returning to the Old Heaven.**

The last three methods are practiced only at advanced levels of spiritual development.

For Whom are Taoist Meditation Techniques Suitable?

In the Western world, it is not easy to find good schools and mentors for this type of meditation. They are more suitable for people who are interested in Taoism, as a philosophy of life, or are engaged in Chinese martial arts such as tai chi.

Qigong

Qigong in Chinese means "work with Qi," work with vital energy. These are complexes of traditional respiratory and physical exercises that arose based on Taoist alchemy and Buddhist psycho-practitioners.

There are thousands of different Qigong practices, including over 80 types of breathing. Medical qigong is a means of preventing and treating disease; In Chinese martial arts communities, qigong is considered an essential component in increasing the fighting abilities of fighters, religion uses meditation practices, and supporters of the practice of Confucianism improve moral qualities.

The qigong master Xu Mingtang, whose grandfather was one of the Shaolin monastery patriarchs, actively promotes this system.

For Whom Qigong Meditations are Suitable

Qigong meditation practices are ideal for those who prefer to integrate ongoing work on the body and energy into the meditation practice. If it is unbearable for you to sit in a static pose for a long time, try Qigong dynamic meditation techniques.

Christian Meditations

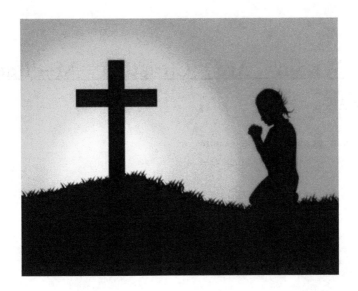

In Eastern traditions, meditation is practiced, as a rule, to calm the mind and achieve enlightenment. In the Christian tradition, the goal of contemplative practice is instead a moral purification, a deep understanding of the Bible, and achieving greater intimacy with God.

Here are some forms of Christian contemplative practice:

- **Contemplative Prayer:** Repetition in whisper or silent prayers or sacred texts.

- **Contemplative reading:** Reading and deep understanding of the Bible.

- **To be with God:** Full awareness of the presence of God with mind, soul, and body.

For Whom Are Christian Meditations Suitable?

It is for those people who believe in God.

Managed Meditations

Guided meditation is a phenomenon in the modern world. It is the easiest way to begin to meditate. You can find a vast number of video and audio meditations on the internet based on various meditative techniques and schools. But after you master the proposed methods, it is recommended that all such moves to independent meditation.

Guided meditation is how to cook with the recipe. You do everything exactly as you say, and at the exit, you get a ready-made, completely edible dish. But once you have mastered the basic principles of cooking, you can cook your meal. It will have a unique, individual taste.

The following types of guided meditations are distinguished:

- **Traditional meditation: It** is an audio or video file with a step-by-step voice guide that gradually brings you into a meditative state.

- **Guided visualization:** In contrast to traditional meditation, it is proposed here to imagine some object, scenery, or journey for deeper reflection and contemplation for relaxation and healing.

- **Relaxation:** This type of guided meditation helps to achieve deep relaxation of the whole body. As a rule, it is accompanied by music or sounds of nature. The purpose of this technique is to relax and find peace.

Affirmations: This type of meditation is used to fix a thought in mind to tune oneself to a specific wave.

Who Can Adopt Guided Meditation?

Guided meditations are suitable for those who find traditional forms of meditation too challenging performing, who want to meditate, but don't know where to start. They can also be useful for performing a specific task, such as increasing self-esteem, relieving tension in the body, and getting rid of pain or resentment.

CONCLUSION

Thank you for reading all this book!

Hypnosis is usually more tedious and can induce sleep. It may be a tool for people who are fighting various sleep disorders, such as insomnia or sleepwalking. For people with insomnia, hypnosis can help the body and mind relax and eliminate the anxiety of being unable to fall asleep.

Insomnia is a difficulty of falling asleep or falling asleep for a long time until you feel refreshed the next morning. Most of us will experience sleep disruption and will know how you feel when you can't seem to fall asleep. Temporary and persistent insomnia are two types of insomnia. Temporary insomnia lasts from one night to three or four weeks. Common causes of transient insomnia include jet lag, changes in daily or working conditions, stress, caffeine, and alcohol. Persistent insomnia lasts for at least four weeks almost every night. Drugs that may be due to pain or medical conditions often disrupt sleep. These may include arthritis, Parkinson's disease, asthma, allergies, hormone changes, or mental health problems.

Many factors can cause insomnia, such as loud noise, uncomfortable bed, drinking too much caffeine or alcohol before going to bed, or sleeping in a room that is too hot or too cold.

There are various methods for the treatment of insomnia. Cognitive-behavioral therapy for insomnia can help you control or eliminate the negative thoughts and behaviors that keep you awake. During long periods of wakefulness, patterns of sleep disturbances may embed in your subconscious mind. Hypnotic sleep can help to solve these problems.

You can improve your sleeping habits. For example, create a routine, exercise regularly, reduce alcohol, caffeine, and nicotine, avoid eating big meals late at night, and place electronic equipment outside the bedroom. You can try hypnosis to treat insomnia if you have a hard time falling asleep, or you have a specific sleep disorder such as restless leg syndrome, night terrors, and sleepwalking.

When you sleep, your body will work hard, which is good for your physical and mental health. Insomnia can have a severe impact on the body. The long-term effects of insomnia are even more critical, leading to poor coordination and decision-making ability, as well as medical conditions such as high blood pressure, diabetes, and thyroid disease. The effects of insomnia on the heart can be dangerous or even fatal. Some of the possible impacts of insomnia on the brain include the inability to concentrate, choking creativity, short-term and long-term memory loss, and mood swings. Other risks of a sleep-deprived brain are hallucinations, mania, impulsive behavior, depression, delusions, and suicidal thoughts.

Positive affirmation is also called happiness affirmation, which will help you build a definite look, which is essential for maintaining positive energy and attracting positive things to your life. Some of the statements are: I like to learn new things, the universe is more significant than my problems, I believe the creator and everything will be elegant, today I can laugh, I choose not to worry, I am healthy and capable of finishing the work, no one can steal my joy, I am enough, I am grateful for everything I have, and I strive to be a better self. Affirmations help you find happiness, which improves health, reduces stress, creates success, protects your heart, strengthens your immune system, and extends your life span.

You have already taken a step towards your improvement.

Best wishes!

Weight Loss Hypnosis Mastery

Positive Affirmations Law of Attraction Meditation for Exercise Motivation, Weight Loss Success, to Quit Sugar & Stop Sugar Cravings, & to Love Your Body

Written By

DAVID JENKINS

INTRODUCTION

Thank you for purchasing this book!

Slow-wave sleep is essential for human health and well-being and the consolidation of memory. This stage of sleep has shown a decrease with age, and this decrease is associated with the development of several neurological diseases. Prescription drugs designed to improve sleep (or more accurately: sedatives) have been shown to reduce slow-wave sleep. These drugs may also have serious adverse side effects and are usually highly addictive. Slow-wave rest (also called deep sleep) is the third stage of the sleep cycle. It is called slow-wave because EEG will show synchronized low-frequency activity at this stage. EEG or electroencephalography uses electrodes placed on the scalp to measure brain activity by detecting electrical changes.

Enjoy your reading!

Sound Meditation

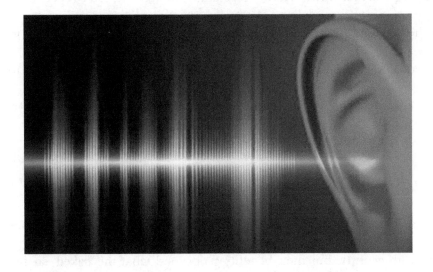

In Western countries, sound meditation is becoming increasingly popular - this is meditation in which harmonious sounds are the object of concentration. Such classes have therapeutic effects thanks to specially selected musical instruments. All of these tools have known since ancient times. Everything new is well forgotten old.

Let's find out the sounds of which instruments can help us in healing diseases.

Singing Bowls

Singing Tibetan bowls emit a resonant, healing tone. However, not all dishes created with the proper level of customization. Therefore, it is essential to find the right meal that you feel good. Choosing the right tool is a crucial factor. If the sound of the bowl significantly improves your well-being, then the instrument suits you.

Fork

These small metal forks have helped musicians tune their instruments since the 18th century, but their benefits go beyond what the naked ear feels. Like singing bowls, tuning forks make a sound when struck.

You can listen, absorb good vibrations, or apply tuning forks in some regions of the body, especially in energy centers or at meridian lines. It's believed that this is a great way to release energy blocks in the body and initiate a psychological reaction that helps relieve pain.

The Music of the Wind

Shamans often use rattling tools to tune into animal archetypes, connect with the spiritual world, and drive out the disease. It is not unusual for a shaman or healer to beat a tambourine over a client's body or drum I during a spiritual journey. In particular, the singing sticks of wind music are of mysterious origin, but their calming effect cannot deny.

Singing Mantras

The singing of mantras is often included in yogic practices, enhancing the psychological effect of asanas, and promoting a more reliable connection between the mind and body. Using your voice for healing is an intimate, in-depth experience that allows you to get a powerful spiritual discharge.

Most of us can chant because not everyone can sing. And even when we cannot use our voice, merely repeating the mantra in mind can produce surprisingly strong results.

It is not surprising that yogis and meditators specially arrange immersion sessions in sound. It is easy, affordable, friendly, and helpful. By merely singing, drumming, or resonating singing bowls, we can improve our mood

and reduce stress.

Benefits of Incorporating Meditation into your Work

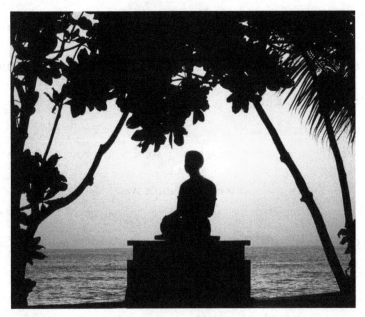

1. Relax your Brain and Stabilize your Mental State

Meditation helps in parasympathetic dominance and relaxation. It helps maintain the mental state. Busy business people are always sympathetic dominating and may be stressful. Yes, meditation can help with that transition.

2. Concentration and Productivity are Improved

Improving focus and productivity has received particular attention as an effect of mindfulness and is also known as a reason why Google, Facebook, Yahoo!, etc. adopt mindfulness.

3. Free yourself from Anxiety and Sleeplessness and Become a Positive Thinking

It can expect to be effective in reducing anxiety, depression, and stress. There is also a theory that sleep at night improves.

4. Your Intuition Will Sharpen, and you Will be Able to Grasp the Essence of Each Thing

Meditation is said to improve your intuition because it calms your thoughts and increases your sensitivity. It allows you to understand the nature of things and have good ideas and senses at work. You will be able to get the job done.

5. Be Confident in Yourself and Realize your New Potential

"In the "Mindfulness Meditation Method for Brain Performance" by Masao Yoshida, President of the Mindfulness Meditation Society, when you develop your concentration, you will concentrate on what you need to do and stop doing what you need to do. It explained that self-confidence increased and that training that objectively views one's thoughts and feelings will enable one to realize a life of one's own.

``Meditation and mindfulness can make you more confident, and if you're stuck with something, you'll be able to discover new possibilities and open your way."

Other Benefits of Meditation

The Benefits of Meditation for Mental Health

Most people are probably familiar with the positive effects of meditation on mental health: an increased sense of awareness, clarity of mind, compassion, and a sense of calm.

Increased focus is another advantage usually associated with meditation. In one study, it proved that four weeks of daily meditation could increase the level of concentration by 14%, another experiment showed that after the first lesson, "soaring in the clouds" is reduced by 22%.

But these are far from all the benefits of meditation. Researchers at Johns Hopkins University have found that standard meditation programs can alleviate the psychological symptoms of depression, anxiety, and stress-related pain. A published study by Google and Roche, during which their employees meditated daily for eight weeks, yielded similar results: participants reported a 46% decrease in depression and 31% anxiety.

And that is not all. Another study published in the journal PLOS One found that 30 days of meditation increased mental stability by 11%. Moreover, people who meditated for only ten days increased their life satisfaction by 7.5%. Just a few minutes of regular daily meditation helps improve your health - this is enough to relax, breathe, and recharge.

Physical Benefits of Meditation

For appreciating the severe physical benefits of meditation, it is essential to understand how much damage chronic stress can do to the body. Pressure acts on the sympathetic nervous system, causing an influx of natural stress hormones (such as adrenaline and cortisol) into the bloodstream, which can negatively affect the body. For example, too much epinephrine (i.e., adrenaline) can increase the risk of heart attacks and strokes. High levels of cortisol increase blood sugar, suppress the immune system, and narrow blood vessels. Ultimately, intermittent bursts of stress hormones can lead to increased blood pressure, heart rate and cholesterol levels, impaired immunity, energy balance, and sleep quality.

On the contrary, if the body and mind are relaxed, whether, through meditation or other techniques, the parasympathetic nervous system is stimulated as a result of which the body ceases to secrete stress hormones. Many people who meditate regularly have learned to relax "on-demand" and, according to research, can more effectively deal with stress.

A study at the University of California, Davis, found that people who used general meditation programs had lower cortisol levels. A study in 2018 found that medical students who used meditation apps for just ten days had a 12% reduction in stress. Another study found that people who used meditation apps for 30 days reduced their stress level by one third.

Why is stress relief so significant? Due to this, blood pressure, heart rate, and oxygen consumption reduced, which leads to an increase in energy levels, strengthening immunity, and improving sleep. Also, stress reduction is a critical factor in reducing the physical symptoms of many diseases. Take, for example, inflammation associated with stroke, heart disease, cancer, diabetes, and other serious illnesses.

According to a Harvard study, meditation can weaken the genes involved in the inflammatory process and contribute to the development of genes that affect DNA stability.

The Emotional Benefits of Meditation

The brain is that area of our body in which meditation can do real miracles. When we meditate and learn to perceive elevated emotions as passing states, we undoubtedly become more resistant to negative emotions. But one of the most important benefits of meditation is that it can change our way of thinking and thinking and physically change our brain by reprogramming it into more positive thoughts and emotions.

Dark Side of Meditation

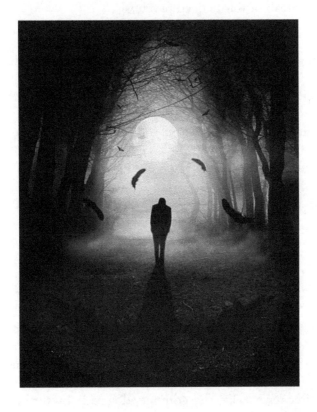

The dark side of meditation: in which cases the development of awareness can lead to a psychological crisis.

Meditation today is presented as a universal tool for mental improvement, which will make the world a better place - it will save us from negative emotions, excessive stress, and the pursuit of consumer pleasures. But meditation has a dark side but not explained well. Instead of calm and pacification, meditation can cause a range of negative experiences and even provoke an outbreak of full-fledged psychosis.

After a 10-day vipassana meditation retreat, 25-year-old American Megan Vogt ended up in a psychiatric clinic. Her parents had to take her from the meditation center - she did not get behind the wheel herself. It seemed to her that the surrounding people her were her psychological projections. She could not distinguish reality from imagination and said that she had to die.

Before trying meditation, Megan suffered from anxiety disorder and took medication, but was never <u>suicidal</u>. After treatment in the clinic, she came to a relatively stable state, but she always thought about what happened at the retreat. After ten weeks, she committed suicide by throwing herself from a bridge.

<u>What is the "Dark Night of the Soul"</u>

It is a rare but by no means the only cause of a psychological crisis that has occurred after intense meditation. In the academic literature, which mentioned recently, but in the Buddhist tradition, such problems are well known and documented.

In one of the sutras, there are lines about monks who go crazy and commit suicide after meditating on mortality. No one said enlightenment is easy.

As the Buddhist teacher and psychologist Jack Kornfield wrote, if you have not encountered pain and fears, you have not yet begun to meditate. Typically, these experiences are considered one of the stages on the path to enlightenment. The most difficult of these stages is the "dark night of the soul," during which a person realizes the illusory nature of his own "I" and the voidness of everything—awareness of this truth accompanied by fear, despair, and psychological struggle.

Once I had an intense "night" that lasted nine months. I experienced despair, panic attacks, loneliness, paranoia, and auditory hallucinations. I could not usually communicate with my family and scrolled thoughts of death continuously in my head.

Modern meditation has long been separated from Buddhism and is perceived by many as a harmless practice - something like morning exercises for the mind. How can you harm yourself simply by sitting and observing your thoughts or breathing?

Usually, nothing horrible happens - you can meditate for years and never experience anything

The benefits of meditation practice explained well in the scientific literature: meditation helps in the treatment of depression and anxiety disorder, relieves stress, facilitates inflammatory reactions, and can improve concentration, memory, and creative thinking. But for some, the secular version of meditation is not only beneficial but also a lot of psychological problems.

What Science Knows about crises in spiritual Practice?

Psychologist Willoughby Britton of Brown University studies the dark aspects of meditation. During practice in a psychiatric clinic, she met two patients who were in the hospital after a retreat. She fell into meditation retreat herself and also experienced severe states.

I thought I was crazy. I thought I was having a nervous breakdown. I mean, I had no idea why all of a sudden, all of this happens to me - for example, why I feel great horror. And only much later did I find out that these are classical states that manifest themselves at certain stages of meditation, which I learned in such a sad way.

Britton decided to study in detail these problematic conditions. Together with her colleagues, she launched a project called "The Diversity of Meditative Experience," in 2017, she published the first final article. Almost each of the more than 100 respondents to the study repeatedly experienced "undesirable conditions" during meditation.

These conditions are increased sensitivity to light, loss of physical sensations, decreased or increased emotions, an increasing sense of anxiety, depersonalization, and the living of traumatic events from childhood. Sometimes the adverse "side effects" of meditation last for whole months.

Many meditation centers are aware of these problems and do not allow people with psychiatric diagnoses to retreat. But almost half of the study participants had no history of injuries and mental disorders. Many of them were themselves experienced teachers of meditation - it hardly suits the explanation that they meditated somehow "wrongly." According to one of the early studies of transcendental meditation, more experienced practitioners had more negative consequences than novices.

After the start of the study, several hundred people turned to Britton, suffering from the undesirable effects of meditation. Most often, problems began during an intensive retreat - for example, a course of vipassana, according to the Goenka system. One session usually lasts at least a week, and each day the participants meditate for 10 hours. They can't talk, look into each other's eyes, write, read, and use them. For many, such a course becomes a liberating experience. For others, it all ends up much worse.

Even the Dalai Lama admits that meditation must be handled carefully: "Westerners go too deep meditation too quickly: they need to learn about Eastern traditions and exercise more than they usually do. Otherwise, mental and physical difficulties arise."

But to experience these difficulties, it is not necessary to go on a retreat. Problems can occur even after using mobile applications such as Headspace.

How Meditation Became Mainstream, and what's Wrong?

Mindfulness meditation arose in the USA in the 1970s as an application of the Zen meditation and the vipassana system. Molecular Biology Specialist John Kabat-Zinn threw away from meditation everything associated with the religious and mystical - gongs, incense, mantras, and worship of Buddha statues. He opened his clinic, where he helped ordinary Americans become more stress-resistant and better cope with their work responsibilities.

In the UK, awareness-raising programs were considered at the legislative level. Everyone meditates office workers, police, house-wives, military, prisoners, teachers, schoolchildren, business people, and movie stars.

The generation of beatniks and hippies through meditation, yoga, and psychedelics sought to awaken cosmic consciousness and world peace. Fifty years later, fund manager David Ford describes the benefits of meditation: "I have become much calmer in responding to volatile markets."

People continuously hear that meditation brings concentration, joy, and love. As a result, they are not ready for what they find in their subconscious mind, chaos, despair, and fear. According to Willoughby Britton, the main reason for concern is the silence of the problem. The modern "mindfulness movement" focuses primarily on the positive effects of meditation on everyday life - stress relief, increased concentration, and performance.

But meditation is a powerful tool for exploring your mind, not a way of complacency. As one of the leading researchers of mindfulness, Richard Davidson, notes, there are two ways to apply meditation - deep and superficial. The first method aims to change your "I," and characteristics understand the nature of consciousness. The second helps to relax after a hard day, focus on current tasks, and get more pleasure from the little joys of everyday life. But in fact, the border between these two methods is very fragile.

Buddhist meditation is not to make us happier, but to radically change our perceptions of ourselves and the world around us. Therefore, it is not surprising that meditation causes adverse effects - dissociation, anxiety, and depression.

To whom Meditation can Harm

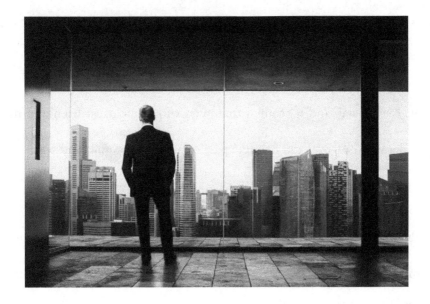

Research is just beginning to be conducted, so answering this question is still difficult. One thing that can be said more or less confidently: is that the adverse effects of meditation cause the same mechanisms that make it useful.

Thanks to the research of neurophysiologists, we know quite well how meditation practices affect the brain. First of all, it strengthens the prefrontal cortex, responsible for attention and controls the limbic system.

As a result, we begin to track our emotions better - they cease to control our behavior.

For people with increased impulsivity, this is good. But sometimes control becomes too strong: people stop to feel emotions in general, as if this function turns off.

I became asocial, and it seemed that even with my closest friends, I now shared a vast chasm. I did not feel part of anything human and was afraid that it would always be so.

Meditation teaches you to observe your thoughts and emotional states from the side. Many people manage to use this ability to their advantage. But for those prone to dissociative personality disorders, meditation can cause a psychological crisis.

The split between the "participating self" and the "observing self," which is one of the goals of meditation, in psychiatry is considered a symptom of several mental illnesses.

Deep meditation raises suppressed memories, emotions, and feelings from the bottom of the psyche. Some are not ready for this. It is an intricate therapeutic work, which is best done together with a specialist. If you are in a retreat that you cannot even talk to, memories of a traumatic experience can lead to repeated trauma. The advice that they usually give - "just calm down and continue to meditate" - does not help, but can lead to even deeper violations.

Meditation causes an additional release of serotonin - a neurotransmitter that controls many-body systems. It usually contributes to a sense of calm and happiness, and also helps with mild depression. But sometimes excess serotonin can be very worrying - in the same way, some antidepressants act.

As a result, instead of relaxing, a person feels a fit of fear or a panic attack. In people prone to schizophrenia, meditation, in some cases, can cause psychosis.

Now psychologists are developing specialized meditation courses that take into account the characteristics of the human psyche. Moderate meditation combined with psychotherapy can help treat schizophrenia and post-traumatic disorder.

Meditation studies often exaggerate the positive aspects of this practice. Large meta-analyses show that many of these studies are based on a very shaky basis and contain many shortcomings: small sample sizes, lack of a control group, and statistical errors. Scientists usually focus on one positive aspect of meditation and do not ask participants about side effects. The result is a distorted impression that meditation is always and always helpful.

"Now there is such a dogma regarding meditation: if it does not work, then its limitations are still not paid attention to," says Willoughby Britton. "We are told that we did not practice properly. But perhaps this is not a matter of man or practice. The truth of human existence is that there is no such thing that works for everyone."

Meditation is a powerful tool for researching and changing the human psyche. For many people, meditation can be beneficial. But we still have a poor understanding of how this practice works, so you need to be careful and responsive.

Meditation and Power of Mind

In meditation, the mind sinks deeply into itself, but then something throws you out. Deep impressions, thoughts come up, and the depth is already lost. Over time, you repeat this process and find that the character is changing your whole nature. That is the power of meditation.

Meditation occurs when thoughts subside. One way or another, thoughts arise, and you are already in their whirlpool.

Meditation and Unpleasant Memories

Memory can make you sad or enlightened. How often does your mind chew on unpleasant memories?

- "He said such and such."

- "She was so arrogant."

- "They did me something."

Meditation will help your memory switch - you can let go of everything small, insignificant, and remember your infinite nature.

Let go of Thoughts and Desires

Through the mind constantly flowing thoughts. You can cling to your ideas, not allowing them to leave freely - this way, the plate sticks when the player's needle gets stuck. Let the thoughts go. Feel that they are not yours. When you get stuck on one idea, one desire - it causes torment. Meditation occurs when the stream of thoughts subsides.

With the help of meditation, you calm your mind, and then continue to engage in other activities. It is not easy to remain untouched by everyday life, but it will come with the regular practice of meditation. It will become easier. Drop all efforts - to stop thoughts, to concentrate, or to transgress to contemplation.

Go Beyond your Thoughts through Meditation

Meditation is the release of anger and events from the past and planning for the future. Meditation is the acceptance of the present moment; each moment's living is total in its entire depth.

Just understanding this and a few days of continuous practice can change the quality of your life.

Rest during meditation is more profound than the most in-depth and sincerest sleep, which is only possible because you go beyond all thoughts and desires during meditation. It brings incredible calm to the brain. It is similar to the overhaul of the entire body-mind complex.

Meditation -Strength of Mind and Body Health

An everyday maelstrom of events turns your life into a routine, and an avalanche of information does not allow you to relax and distract from the chaos in your thoughts? Meditation is the right decision to find harmony and tranquility.

Numerous studies have shown that those who practice regular meditation for several minutes a day (even if not at a professional but an amateur level) become less anxious and disciplined. Meditation helps restore health, minimize stress, and become happier. These are some arguments in favor of why meditation is required to enter your daily routine.

Reason 1. Meditation Restores Brain Cells

This conclusion was reached by Harvard scientists in 2011. Thanks to the magnetic resonance imaging results, it was possible to find out that meditation affects changes in the gray matter of the brain. The eight-week meditation period activated the regeneration of brain cells, improving memory, learning ability, and concentration.

Reason 2. Meditation Reduces the Risk of Cardiovascular Disease

Scientists, Schneider, and Grim conducted a study in which 201 people with ischemia participated. Half of the subjects practiced regular meditation practices, while others led a simple lifestyle. After five years, the meditation group showed a 48 percent reduction in the risk of heart attack and heart attack!

Reason3. Meditative Techniques Reduce Anxiety and Depression

Scholars Goyal and Singh found that constant meditation helps to better deal with pain and depression. Fadel Zeidan, a neuroscientist at Wake Forest University (USA), conducted a similar study. He demonstrated that meditation activates areas of the brain that are responsible for behavioral control and processing of emotions. Meditation reduces conscious perception by 40%, pain level by 70%, and associated discomfort by 40%.

Reason 4. Meditation Strengthens the Immune System and Increases the Body's Stamina

Stress and inability to control emotions can provoke various psycho-emotional disorders and somatoform diseases. Your body may feel bad on a physical level, although there may not be any evidence of this. A study from the Harvard Medical School of Medicine proved the activation of energy production in the mitochondria of cells, which improves immunity and stress resistance.

Reason 5. Meditation Fights a Lack of Sleep

Meditation makes your schedule smooth, contributes to faster falling asleep, and better recovery of the body during sleep. The University of Kentucky has published a fantastic study, according to which regular meditation reduces the need for sleep and improves its quality.

Reason 6. Meditation Improves Breathing

Most types of meditation focus on proper breathing, during which the most important physiological processes in the body occur. And this is important for well-being and health: deep breath saturates cells better with oxygen and even increases life expectancy. Meditation helps to introduce the practice of proper breathing into life and develop the habit of breathing deeply, not just in yoga classes.

Reason 7. Meditation Techniques Exacerbate Tactile Sensations

The German scholars of the Ruhr University (Bochum) and the University of Ludwig-Maximillian (Munich), in support of this argument, provided the experience of Zen monks, who proved that meditation develops sensitivity. Finger meditation increased tactile perception by 17%.

Reason 8. Meditation Allows you to Understand yourself, To Establish a Connection with the Inner World

An activist who has dedicated his life to changing the educational program, Will Stanton, in his book The Revolution of Education, suggests introducing meditation as a separate subject. He is sure that meditation helps find the meaning of life and a way out of the most complicated situations, to find peace and tranquility. It is the meditation that directs one to a life goal, helps the younger generation cope with a difficult transitional period, minimizes stress, and avoid mental illnesses.

A gift of awareness like meditation will be beneficial in any case. Exercising regularly, people observe positive changes. They learn to be calm, attentive, sensitive, and all of the above studies are only confirmation of this.

Meditation for the Mind: How to "Pump Up" the Brain

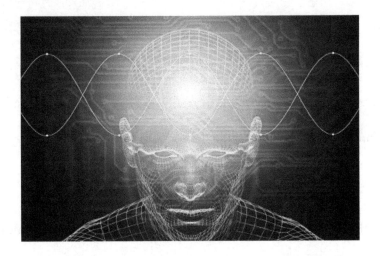

A group of American researchers who investigated the brains of meditating people with magnetic resonance imaging concluded that some regions of the brain in people who regularly meditate are significantly more developed than usual.

Specifically, the "meditators" demonstrated significantly increased volumes of the hippocampus (a region involved in the formation of emotions and memory).

"It is known that people who are constantly meditating, increase the ability to" cultivate "positive experiences, gain greater emotional stability," says Eileen Luders, one of the authors of the study. "The observed differences in brain anatomy can explain why this happens." We add that experienced "meditators" acquire other useful abilities; they reduce stress levels and strengthen the immune system. Nevertheless, the effect of meditation on the brain's structure is a topic that has so far been little studied.

In their work, Lüders and colleagues studied 44 volunteers, of whom half were ordinary people, and a half spent a considerable amount of time doing some form of traditional meditation practice - for example, vipassana. The duration of classes ranged from 5 to 46 years, averaging 24 years. All the "meditators" have confirmed that deep concentration is an essential part of their spiritual practice, and most of them do this for 10 to 90 minutes daily.

Studying the brains of volunteers with the help of MRI, scientists applied two approaches. One consisted of dividing the brain into regions and comparing their characteristics and the other in examining different brain tissues and comparing the amounts of gray matter in one or another of its areas. It was in such ways that both an increase in the volumes of some regions of the brain and an increase in the content of gray matter in the orbitofrontal cortex, thalamus, and temporal lower gyrus were shown. Moreover, there were no cases where representatives of the non-meditating control group would have an advantage over the "meditators" in this.

Since all the areas that meditation effects are related to the emotional life of the brain, Luders believes that there are quite severe neurological changes behind the high degree of emotional control that is developed during meditation practices. "However, it is unknown," she says, "what correlations between them lie at the microscopic, cellular level, and this is worth exploring in the next step." For example, it would be interesting to know whether meditation leads to an increase in the number of neurons, or their sizes, or the appearance of unique additional connections between them.

Note that the study in question was not long-term. So there is still the possibility that the "meditators" who participated in it initially, had larger sizes and a higher saturation of gray matter in some regions of the brain. Maybe this is what made them engage in meditative practice.

It is also worth noting that increased brain volumes do not necessarily mean an "increased mind." For example, dolphins with an unusually large brain do not differ in the extraordinary intelligence that we are accustomed to attributing to them. Read: "Stupid big brain."

Overweight and Obesity

Overweight and obesity are the results of abnormal or excessive body fat that can be harmful to your health. Body Mass Index (BMI) is a simple ratio of body weight to height, often used to diagnose obesity and overweight in adults. The index is calculated as the ratio of body weight in kilograms to the square of growth in meters (kg / m2).

Adults

According to the WHO, the diagnosis of "overweight" or "obesity" in adults is made in the following cases:

- Body Mass Index more than or equal to 25 – overweight.

- Body Mass Index, more than or equal to 30, is obesity.

- Body mass index is the most convenient measure for assessing the level of obesity and overweight in a population since it is the same for both sexes and all age categories of adults. However, BMI should be considered an approximate criterion, as, in different people, it can correspond to a varying degree of completeness.

- In children, when determining excess weight and obesity, age should be considered.

Children Under Five years Old

In children under the age of 5 years, overweight and obesity are defined as follows:

- **Overweight**: If the ratio "body weight/height" exceeds the median value indicated in the Standard indicators of physical development of children (WHO), more than two standard deviations.

- **Obesity**: If the ratio "body weight/height" exceeds the median value indicated in the Standard indicators of physical development of children (WHO), more than three standard deviations;

Charts and tables: WHO standard signs for the physical development of children under five years old - in English.

Children Aged 5 to 19 Years

In children aged 5 to 19 years, overweight and obesity are defined as follows:

- **Overweight**: If the ratio of "BMI / age" exceeds the median value specified in the Standard indicators of physical development of children (WHO), more than one standard deviation.

- **Obesity**: If the ratio of "BMI / age" exceeds the median value indicated in the Standard indicators of physical development of children (WHO), more than two standard deviations.

Charts and tables: WHO standard indicators for the physical development of children and adolescents aged 5-19 years.

Affirmations to Help You Find Happiness

They say that our thoughts are the most potent force in the universe because they can change our lives, enhance our self-esteem, self-love, and add a lot of good energy to us. We are our ideas, and our thoughts translate into words. That is the so-called law of attraction, meaning that no matter what we focus on, we will attract ourselves to life.

Therefore, if you have been focusing on negative thoughts, then you will only attract negative things into your life, even without realizing it. For example, the more you focus on the fact that you are suffering because there is nothing in your life, the longer you stay in that state. However, if you focus on positive thinking, also known as happy thinking, then your subconscious mind will attract more positive things and positive attitudes into your life. For example, if you are grateful for what you already have, and are confident that you can achieve great achievements in life, then the universe will help you achieve this goal.

In summary, if you remain positive and optimistic anyway, and always see all the right things, you will attract more happiness and positivity in your life. Happy people know that the secret of a happy life includes the following elements: embracing every day, embracing every change, engaging in active self-talk, and the most crucial link-positive affirmation of happiness and success.

Positive affirmation, also known as happiness affirmation, will help you build a definite look, which is essential for maintaining positive energy and attracting positive things to your life. Through learning and applying statement, you will learn to control your happiness and dreams! All you need to do is read the following list of positive affirmations, in which you will find inspiring morning affirmations, daily affirmations, and love affirmations.

After choosing your favorite person, you can write some positive affirmations on the paper and spend a few minutes reading them aloud every day (preferably in front of the mirror). Also, you can repeat this process several times a day to get better results. Now, reading does not mean reading them like a newspaper. You need to feel every word of your affirmation, accept it, and imagine it vividly! You need to believe in what you say with all your heart because believing means striving for your happiness and realizing your dreams.

I Choose to Be Happy Today

Today is a brand-new day, and happiness is an excellent choice. Anyone can choose pain and anger. Choosing happiness requires strength and confidence. Today, I can use my joy to change the world!

Who Am I?

That is not a problem for me; every part of me is perfect. I can accomplish what others cannot do because I am me. I don't need to compare myself with other people, nor do I feel that I am inferior to others. They are them, and I am me. Today is the secret—I being me, which is a good thing!

People Are Not Sure Who I Am

Others have opinions about who I am, but they do not define me. I am the person I choose and the person I want to be. And I will not accept any negative thoughts about me or change for others. If they are not satisfied with me, I can tell them, thank you, no, thank you. I will define myself.

I Like to Learn New Things

This positive affirmation reminds you of the exciting prospect of learning new things today. I'm curious and smart, and I can study hard. When faced with challenges, I will not flinch. I can work hard and learn everything.

I Am Free

I can live freely without worrying or worrying. I got rid of the mistakes of the past. I can voluntarily become the person who the universe makes me. Licensing is self-sufficient so as not to feel unworthy. I don't have the opinions of others, and they didn't make me. Most importantly, I got rid of doubters and haters who didn't understand my life. Today, I am free to be me!

The Universe is Bigger than My Problem

Today, the earth has not lost control. My Creator is here; more significant than any problems I have today. The universe cares about me. Therefore, I can connect with nature and appreciate all the beauty that is much bigger than me.

My Contribution is Important to Me and Others

This positive is undoubtedly a valuable reminder. I have something to share with my world. The people around me, no matter how much they look, need my contribution. If I flinch, someone will fail. My thoughts are firm, and I can solve the problem. People need my gifts. I will be full of confidence and goals.

I Believe the Creator, and Everything Will Be Fine

It is a good thing to trust the Creator. I don't need crutches; I need a supernatural, omnipotent person to put the stars in place. He is bigger than the world, more significant than the doubters. He is by my side, and I have full confidence in him because he uses me to do great things today.

Today I Can Laugh

This motto tells us—laughter is always the best medicine. Therefore, I will laugh for my soul and accept its beneficial health medicine. I will laugh at things that I cannot control. I will laugh at something that I can control. I will laugh at my weaknesses, mistakes, and humanity. Laughter trumps pain and pessimism about life. I won't let the fear dealer tell me to hide and fear life.

I Choose Not to Worry

I won't worry because it will kill people. Worry kills joy. Also, concerns tell me the worst. Fear prevents me from trying. It stole my life: anxiety and boredom. I refuse to worry about things that I cannot control. I will not worry about things that I cannot control. I chose not to suffer because it would not make me better.

I Choose Peace, Do Not Hate

When everything is chaotic around me, I choose to maintain peace. My choice is peace rather than revenge, and I select unity over hatred. I want peace and faith instead of manipulating others. During the visualization, I breathed calmly and exuded fear.

The Creator is Nothing

That is a positive affirmation; thought-provoking. Our creator is more significant than any problems I have encountered. He is greater than any hatred I face. He can stop me from falling. When I cried to him, he heard my voice. No one can keep me away from his love and protection. For him, it is not difficult to accomplish anything in my life.

I'm not Perfect, and It Doesn't Matter

Perfect for sunset, not for people. No one is perfect, no matter what they tell you. There is no ideal body, face, brain, or work. Life is a significant imperfect experience, and it doesn't matter. People are imperfect people. I'm so happy that it's not perfect, it will be boring. I can accept my way!

I am Strong and Capable of Finishing Work

I can do whatever I want. I am capable, capable, and work hard to complete the work. No one can take it away from me, and I am stronger than yesterday and healthier tomorrow. I will finish the work according to my schedule.

I Cannot Accept Others

I accept the imperfections of others. I will not let them fail or disappoint me. That's their business, not me, and I don't need them to succeed in finding my peace or joy. I will not rely on others to find my happiness. If they disappoint me, I will still accept them. I am a lovely person, even if the people around me are not.

My love for others does not depend on their behavior. I don't love what others do for them, but who they are. If they fail, get angry and even yell at me, I don't have to be sad. They did not define my love for them. I can love but be firm. I can set boundaries for them, and this is a thing full of love. Finally, I can correct them, which is also a thing whole of love. Keeping quiet and ignoring their bad behavior is not love, but hateful. I will stand up for myself that is love. This positive affirmation will make you rest assured that you will give respect to famous people.

I'm making Progress, and It Doesn't Matter

Today, I may fail. I may spend a lot of time. Yes, because I am in Progress. Today, I will grow and change, and when I make mistakes, I will learn. I will bear my mistakes and be responsible for my errors. The most certain thing is that I will not be trivial; I will be secure, do not worry about messing up. We learn from our failures—this is the key to your rebound! Even if there are any difficulties, I will not give up. If the situation becomes difficult today, I will not give up. I will never allow self-pity or self-blame games. I can do challenging things. I can take a moment to complete the task in front of me. I will do what I need to do in the way I want to do.

Most importantly, when someone tells me I can't do it, I won't give up. When someone says that are better than me, I will not give up. Maybe it is right, but I will not give up the efforts to improve myself and the world around me.

My Creativity

Today, I can use my creativity. I can find a unique solution to the problem. I can think outside the box. My creativity looks different from other people's creativity. I may not be an artist, but I can paint something inspiring. Although I may not be a musician, I can sing to comfort someone. In the end, I may not be a writer, but I can write a letter to encourage sick friends. I am very creative and exceptional for me.

No One Can Steal My Joy

My joy is safe. It does not depend on the acceptance or understanding of me by others. It also doesn't depend on how many likes I get in the latest social media posts or how many followers I have. My happiness does not base on others, but on me—and me alone. My joy is safe because it cannot take away!

The Universe is good for me

When you feel uncomfortable, it isn't easy to believe that the universe will support you and stand by your side. However, this is what you need to do. Always remember that the universe is right for you. Believe it and repeat it once a day until it becomes part of you because that is the only truth. The universe has been working hard to bring you joy, happiness, and all the positive things you deserve. All your dreams will become a reality one day—you need to believe it.

I'm enough

You are enough, and you deserve it. There is no need to worry about achieving specific achievements in life. Things do not define you. You are enough to meet your needs, and you need to believe it.

I Should Be Healthy, Happy and Successful

If you think you should be healthy, happy, and prosperous, then you will. However, if you do not do this, the universe will have difficulty understanding your information. It would help if you believed that you deserve to have the great things in life, because by doing so, you will deliver positive vibrations to the universe, and the world will reward you with higher positivity. All of this is to build a concrete foundation, thereby attracting more positive emotions for your life.

My heart is always willing to accept and accept all forms of love. To get precious happiness and blessings, you also need to be prepared to pay. Your heart needs to be open and give and receive love in various forms. You need to live out love. An open mind and an open mind life is the first step to attract more love and more positive things to your life. It is essential to find a balance, which will be the cornerstone of future success and happiness.

I am Grateful for Everything I Have

When giving positive affirmation of success and Happiness, being grateful for everything you already have is one of the most important things, because thanksgiving itself is a definite form. Therefore, you don't have to focus on what you don't have and want to have. Instead, it would help if you concentrate on thanking you for what you already have because it will put you in a more positive state, which is the core of prosperity and Happiness. Happiness is my innate right. I earn all the good things in life.

It would help if you believed that happiness is your birthright, not something impossible. You should be happy, and you should have all the goodness in life! You can prove to yourself and others that you deserve to be respected, loved and appreciated without climbing a mountain. You already have all of them. You need to find it and hug it!

Daily Recognition of Happiness and Success

If you already believe that your life is full of Happiness, peace, blessings, and love, then you will live such an experience. Remember, everything comes from your thoughts and ideas. You are, you become your idea. Therefore, please feel free to believe and believe that your life is full of the greatest things in the universe, and the world will work harder with your support.

I Strive to Be a Better Self

Always focus on improving your habits and investing energy to be better, bigger, and more reliable. It would help if you worked hard to be a better self because this is the only way to return all the good things in life. The universe needs to know that you are doing your best to realize your potential.

I Will Choose Happiness, Anyway

That is my favorite and one of the most complicated. When life disappoints you, it isn't easy to choose to stay happy anyway, but it is necessary. Why? Because the primary purpose of every challenge and every hardship is to make you stronger, more resilient, and smarter. When unfortunate things happen, instead of living in pain, it is better to choose to get out of trouble and decide to be happy regardless of everything.

Happiness Inspires Me

Believe that happiness is the only cure for your soul and the single dominant force that can invigorate your spirit. Live Happiness, imagine Happiness, and be excited about all the little things that are so significant. The core of true happiness is to live every day as if this is your last day because it will happen one day. When you believe that your natural state is composed of happiness and unconditional love, you will start living like this, and you will begin to attract more positive things to your life.

That is to be grateful for what you have, believe in the greatness you deserve, and show what you already have. That is the only secret to attracting a lot of happiness and success in daily life.

I Believe in my Intuition

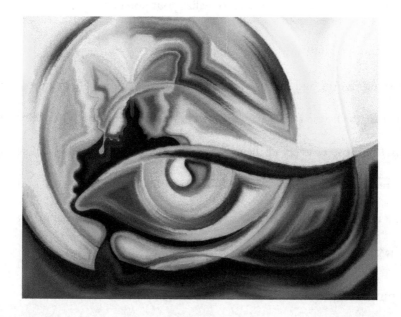

The intuition is that there is only a small voice in your head that can tell you when something went wrong or when it was right. When making decisions, you need to believe in this voice, and you need to think that it will help you make informed decisions and protect you from all the negative factors in your life. The most significant source of negative emotions is that everyone around you is planning something that is not good for you or is jealous of your success.

It would help if you got along with positive people who believe in you whole heartedly and are happy about your success. And, it would help if you keep reminding yourself, because the more you think about it, the more positive people in the universe will make you enter your life, and they will become your most significant support. The key to success includes the following three words: passion, creativity, and determination.

Passion will fill your life with love. Creativity will ensure that you will never get bored, and determination will give you the ability to move on even if you think you will not. If you practice this affirmative attitude several times a day, your work, hobbies, and everything you do will be significantly improved, and you will achieve significant achievements, which will undoubtedly receive attention and receive corresponding rewards.

- I am happy and content with the present.
- The universe is doing everything it can bring me complete happiness.
- I will only attract happy and positive people.
- I will naturally like those things and people who support my complete happiness and peace.
- Happiness is an inherent right.
- No matter how I am, I will choose happiness.

- Happiness is one of my most important values. All my decisions are consistent with bringing me a complete sense of joy.

- I choose happiness every day instead of any other emotions.

- When I feel unhappy, I immediately choose to feel happy and satisfied.

- I can completely control my emotions, including happiness.

- Happiness is so beautiful because it is my nature, and this is what I think about every day.

- Apart from determining and controlling my level of happiness, no one can do it.

- I take full responsibility for my happiness level.

- My skin is great.

- I am satisfied with my identity and accept myself wholly and completely.

- I only keep positive and happy thoughts and only allow them.

- I look at life optimistically, full of vitality every day.

- I bath with universal happiness and love.

- No matter where I am, I will only see the smiles and happiness among the people around me.

- My peaceful nature inspires people and changes their mood, and makes me feel better.

- The more I love, the happier I will be. That is why I choose to enjoy every day.

- Optimism and happiness run through my veins.

- I see happiness in every pore.

- God wants me to be happy and supports me to pursue it every day.

- I know that when I put in more work and seek self-growth, I become happier. That is why I grow up every day.

- Happiness comes from my heart, not from the outside.

- I meditated and prayed for happiness, which brought me more joy and satisfaction.

- I am full of joy every day.

- I like to bring happiness to others because I know it will make me happier. That is a win-win situation.

- My happiness and infinite degree make me smile.

- I love myself because this is pure happiness.

- I have behaved like a child all my life, entirely accepted, full of curiosity in life, full of happiness and vitality.

- No matter where I go, happiness will follow.

- I see life in a way that I can only live once, so any unhappy moments waste time.

- No matter what others say about me, I will always be happy and love myself.

- Happiness and love are the main motivations of my life.

- I know I focus on expansion, so that's why I only focus on happiness and love.

- All my experiences made me completely ecstatic.

- I quickly eat proper food and do vigorous exercise, which makes me feel lively and healthy to create happiness in me.

- Happiness is my definition of people, not anyone else.

- Every morning when I get up, I will thank the person I love, which makes me feel happy.

- I will forgive others quickly, and I won't hold grudges or resentments because I know this will hinder my happiness.

- I meditate on happiness every day, and it brings more joy into my life.

- My focus is on energy flow. That is why I chose to focus only on the things that are good for my happiness.

- I enjoy my happiness and never feel in it.

- I let go of some ideas that were useless to my life or hindered my happiness.

- I can be sure that happiness is that I keep looking for it because I will find what I want.

- No matter what I have done in the past, I should still get and choose happiness.

- I am not reflecting on my situation, but on how to choose to respond to the job. I want a reaction that will only benefit my health and happiness.

- Every day I am sure that I feel happy and happy.

- My goal is to be happy and remind myself of this fact all day long.

- I couldn't help meeting people who longed for my happiness.

- I am full of enthusiasm and goals for this life because I know that doing so will make me happier.

- I am engaged in some self-care routines that can help me concentrate, find peace, and rebirth.

- People are always talking about how high my energy is and how I exude happiness and love.

- If someone hinders the happiness of my life, they will naturally get rid of my life quickly.

- I will not tolerate negative people in my life.

- The only thing I know and seek is happiness and love. Everything else is new to me.

- Whenever I choose to do this, I can bring more happiness in life.

- Happy thoughts come naturally and easily.

- Every day I am attracted to situations that fill me with joy.

- I choose to be happy every day.

- Happiness is my innate right.

- I woke up for today's awakening, and I chose happiness.

- My life is full of gratitude and happiness.

- I am grateful for the good things in life.

- Happiness is my choice every day.

- I feel happy, healthy, and grateful.

- I choose happiness and joy every moment.

- Even in difficult times, I choose to see the good in life.

- When I realize all the blessings in my life, I will find that I am naturally happy.

- Happiness is my spiritual alchemy.

- Happiness is a natural response to gratitude.

- Many simple joys in life bring me great happiness.

- I can choose to be happy at any time.

- May all beings, including me, be happy.

- Even when faced with challenges or difficulties, I still choose to be happy.

- My natural state is happiness and joy. I live there.

- I am happy to choose.

- When you ask me why I feel happy, I will answer. Let me count.

- I live a happy, healthy, and harmonious life.

- My life is full of happiness, peace, and love.

- Happiness, health, and harmony are my life.

- My happy life begins now.

- A happy life continually cultivates every day.

- I am happy, I know, so I show it to me.

- The world deserves true happiness.

- Let us live such a life so that our happiness is beneficial to the entire world.

- May my happiness be a gift for my friends and family.

- I am free to choose happiness.

- I am happy to be alive.

- I thank everyone in my life who loves me.

- I thank every opportunity that life has brought me.

- I am grateful for every second in my life.

- Thanksgiving can help me attract more things that need to be thankful.

- Happiness is a part of my life.

- I am happy, successful, and independent.

- I deserve success and wealth.

- I should be happy and enjoy my success.

- Success is something that can help me help others.

- I become more and more successful and happy every day.

- I believe in positive power.

- I believe I will make a favorable decision.

- I can live everything that life shows for me.

- Whenever I choose, I can turn a new page.

- Today I will be happier than yesterday.

- This day will be a happy time.

- I choose happiness over everything.

- I surrounded by peace, harmony, and vitality.

- My inner peace can help me through everything.

- Peace and happiness go hand in hand with me.

- I like to spend some time enjoying the tranquility of the day.

- I attract people who are peaceful and peaceful in life.

- I can shape the ideal reality.

- I create the life I want with good emotion.

- Everything is always good for me.

- When I feel happy, I will show more reasons for happiness.

- I am happy now.

- I accept that joy is my nature.

- I deserve to be happy.

- My joy comes from my heart.

- I take every part of myself through unconditional love to create my happiness.

- Satisfaction is the essence of my existence.

- I have seen many positive aspects of my life.

- I keep creating everything I desire.

- I feel happy in everything I do.

- I am satisfied with myself as a person.

- I allow myself to be happy.

- I make myself feel good.

- The happiness created the life I always dreamed of I choose now.

- The joy of following me reveals the path to the best life.

- I want pleasure to keep me perfectly healthy.

- Everyone around me feels happy.

- I use ecstasy to create the possibility of happiness for others.

- I destined to live a happy life.

- When sharing with others, my inner joy expands.

- All the goodness in my life is that I am willing to find happy results every moment.

- My happiness reflected in everything I attract.

- My inner happiness is the source of all good things in my life.

- I feel happy in everything I do.

I like every moment of the day. I naturally feel relaxed about the things that have troubled me. I am the leader of my life, which makes me feel happy and healthy. No matter how I look or feel, I will choose to be satisfied. I will always be satisfied. I am not afraid of anything in my life, because I have the power of happiness and love, and can eliminate fear anytime, anywhere. I see life as a classroom, where I am always learning new ways of happiness. I am delighted with this human experience.

The angels even stood on my side, supporting me in my pursuit of happiness. I bless the happiness of others because I know that I must bless me. Not only do I pursue happiness, but the more I continue, the more pleasure I will find. Everything in this world is good, I feel safe, and security brings me happiness. My personality radiates joy to the world, and this happiness radiates to me.

The more I understand my happiness, the more I will inspire my lifelong pursuit. People will remember how happy I was and how glad I made them. All I do is do most joyful things in life. I look in the mirror every morning and love myself because I know that when I do this, I feel good about myself, which brings me more happiness. I set ambitious goals for myself because I believe in myself, and by achieving them, I become happier.

I know that it is not my life that makes me happy, but who I am. I chose to look only at the front. I embrace the journey in various ways, shapes, and forms. That makes my life happier. I love happiness; happiness loves me. I now have everything I need to be completely happy. I live a life commensurate with my morals and values, which makes me incredibly tremendous and happy. The clothes I wear make my skin feel good and therefore make me feel happier.

I often detox my body and mind because I know that my body is my temple. If I feel bad, I cannot get the most happiness. I will not be in any negative state for a long time. I made myself think that this is the process. Then I returned to a peaceful state. In the process of marching towards happiness, I am moving fast—more and more every day. Joy and happiness make me feel natural and relaxed. I challenge people's beliefs about their unhappiness because I know my permission and defense will enter my life. Therefore, I encourage others to be happy.

I was lost in the pursuit of happiness and found myself. When I am not satisfied, I love myself. I have complete control over this. That makes me feel happier, and I directly like negative thoughts and feelings. That dissipated them and brought me back to a happy place. I have full confidence in my ability and life, which makes me feel happy. I am the master of destiny, and I have chosen the chance of complete happiness now and in the future. I look back and learn from it. Don't beat yourself or stay in the past. This growth has helped me become more permanently happy.

I smile at strangers on the street and in life because it brings happiness to both of us. I have never allowed making me more comfortable. I quickly showed my spiritual connection and made me feel happier every day. My intuition naturally tells me that I need to do more to be satisfied. I am talented and unique, which makes me feel incredibly happy. I am pleased with everything I have done in this life. I am so glad to have another chance every day to wake up and become more comfortable. I see fantastic opportunities everywhere, which makes me happy. My spirit is always high. Every day I exist, I feel so glad and relieved. I will naturally feel ecstatic.

I am happy to see the happiness of others. Every day I perform random acts of kindness, which brings joy to me and others. I am glad and exuberant all day long. My dreams showed me ways to make myself more comfortable and more peaceful. I took action on them because I knew that my higher self was trying to communicate with me. If my path does not bring me happiness, I will give myself full permission to change my way immediately. In my life, I will not do what makes others happy, but do what makes me happy. When life gives me lemons, I make lemonade. The unexpected mood pleased me.

I am always looking for new activities and new things that want me. I know that a quiet mind makes me feel happy. That is why I often meditate my mind through meditation. I don't think anything makes me feel more comfortable and more active and engages in these activities. I work hard, work hard, which gives me a great sense of balance and happiness. I know my thoughts reflect my reality, which is why I only think happy thoughts revealed in my life.

Ways of Happiness in Life

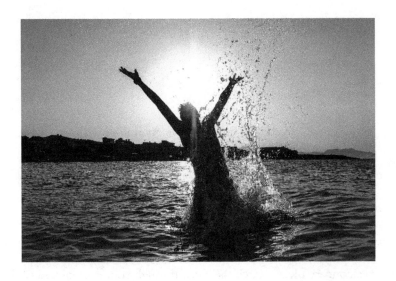

Be Active

When you follow a familiar route, your brain starts daydreaming. It shifts attention from driving to your inner thoughts, which we call wandering. Have you ever experienced it? Walking is a unique feature of human beings. It allows our brain to move away from the task at hand and focus on other things. It helps us improve creativity, but it hinders our ability to live and enjoy the time.

Matt Killing worth is a former researcher at Harvard University. He believes that people want to get rid of many things in life, but they mainly wish to Happiness. It studied our brains and concluded that our wanderings are the cause of our unhappiness. He believes that the influence of the wandering mind on our happiness is more significant than income, education, gender, and marital status.

He has been engaged in scientific research for many years and asked people three

questions:

- What do you think?

- What are you doing?

- Are you thinking about what you are doing?

If people answer "yes" to the last question, then their brains are not present at
this time, and their sense of happiness will reduce. He concluded that existence
is related to Happiness. It seems that the presence is crucial to our Happiness. If
you go to a concert, please watch the show through your eyes instead of through
the camera lens. If you are traveling by road, don't worry about reaching your
destination and enjoy the drive. If you are having dinner with your family, please
ask them questions and listen to their answers. Attend.

Caring, Building Connections, Creating

Humans are social animals. We like to connect with others. We want to take care
of others. With people who care about you, you care about them too. Connect
with old friends. Focus on showing your friends and family that you care about
them, and thank them for their lifetime. Establish more profound connections
with loved ones. The most important job in my life is to be a father and take care
of my family. I try to have dinner with my family every day. I instruct children's

football teams, participate in their karate exercises, and interact with them every day.

I call or text my friends as much as possible. I check my parents every day. I intend to keep in touch with my family, friends, and everyone I contact. Create something by hand; build something. Dan Ariely is one of my favorite behavioral economists, and he emphasizes the importance of creating things with our hands. He believes that creating jobs with our hands will bring us Happiness.

He pointed out that IKEA understands this concept, which is why they sell complex furniture parts with vague instruction manuals and ask customers to assemble them. This process is terrible, but the satisfaction people get after building their furniture is vast. It is fantastic to create things with both hands and bring your inner joy. Stay in touch with the people you care about and create a life worth sharing and starting today.

Celebrate Every Victory

Football players celebrate every game, every tackle and every touchdown. They do not pay attention to the score, but celebrate everything. Take this way of thinking and celebrate every time you complete a task. If you reply to the email, please stop and celebrate. If your conversation with colleagues is confusing, please enjoy your achievements.

Dr. Rick Hanson advises people to taste positive experiences. He encourages people to celebrate after achieving any achievements. This type of exercise will train your brain from a positive state to a positive trait. What are you celebrating today?

Exercise

Exercise increases endorphins and reduces cortisol and epinephrine in the body. It is also an effective treatment for depression and anxiety. According to the New York Times, a small amount of exercise has a significant impact on our Happiness. People who exercise at least once a week are happier than those who do not use it. Tony Robbins believes that sports create emotions. If you don't like how you feel, go to the gym, walk outdoors, or practice yoga. Twelve minutes of exercise can last up to 12 hours.

Sleep

According to the American Psychological Association, more rest will make you happier, healthier, and safer. Based on my experience, I can assure you that a tired person is not a happy person. You need to sleep to work. Sleep is essential for your overall well-being and well-being. Lack of sleep can slow down your reaction time, damage your memory, and reduce your sense of Happiness. It also weakens your immune system and slows your critical thinking. If you want to be happy, please pay attention to the amount and quality of sleep.

Expect Less

Research shows that happy people value satisfaction as their primary motivation. If you are satisfied, you may be satisfied. Working towards realistic goals will cultivate happiness because you pursue things that bring Happiness. The Science and Practice of Open Consciousness" by Loch Kelly: "Evidence shows that 10% of our happiness depends on external success."

Enjoy Work

Happy people like their work. Their pursuit is not money or fame, but the satisfaction they bring. Those who get stuck in an unfinished and profitable job will soon discover that this is not the way to Happiness. Pay paid for your skills, and money is only one aspect of job satisfaction. Pursue your favorite job or occupation. If you have not respected in your work, you will find a job you are satisfied with; I assure you that they exist.

Many people waste their best time and make money for their families while leaving their passions at the same time. However, your happiness is also a top priority. The writer Jonathan Fields pointed out in "How to Live a Good Life": "What about money? That is important. But it is not what you might think. If you live in poverty and cannot afford a basic life, make money. Every dollar you get increases happiness and life satisfaction. However, once your living expenses quickly paid, more money has little effect on Happiness.

Live for Today

Avoid being troubled by previous failures. Everything that has passed away is gone, and reflection on the future will only cause higher pressure and worry. You don't see what will occur next, let alone predict the next step. So, what is the point of concern? Live in the moment and do your best. Focus on the moment, and you will gain a lot, for example, to appreciate the beauty of life and reduce stress.

Wisdom, Freedom from Complacency and Fear": "All in all, happiness does not stem from the goal of happiness, but from being able to appreciate the journey, especially the current experience in our lives."

Choose Happiness

Step by step, re-establish goals and maintain a flexible approach. That requires an open mind and positive thinking. Choose happiness as your primary goal, not overshadow other competitive areas. A point of view does not bind you, and you can always choose a positive attitude. You can accept failure, which is not very helpful for you to be happy or build a favorable opinion. Regardless of your choice, as circumstances change, there will be another day to show your best self.

Embrace change with open attention and lifetime will be better than you think. Writer Jonathan Fields must say: "True happiness does not appear when you choose to be happy, but when you find something that makes you happy and then do it."

Social

Humans are social animals. It is connected to our DNA to communicate with others. Areas in the brain called mirror neurons allow us to recognize and mirror the behavior of other people. That is why yawning is contagious because scientists believe that yawning is a sign of unconscious social connections.

Happiness and love flourish in the company of others, which is essential to your health and Happiness. If you isolate yourself, it is likely to produce negative emotions. In this age of technological connections, people are more isolated and lonelier than ever before, leading to mental health problems.

Cherish those things that are important to you through regular social connections. For example, research shows that married people are happier than single people. It highlights that close ties are essential to your overall emotional health. "Happiness is not a ready-made thing. It comes from your behavior."

Don't Compare Yourself to Others

Ambitiousness is excellent, but jealousy only makes you unhappy. Comparing with others has its limitations. We may have invested too much in the lives of others and lost our journey. Everyone's situation is different. Comparing with others will cause you nothingness and pain. Other people's lives may look perfect, but we are not aware of a hidden story. Although it helps to learn from them, too much competition may destroy your inner peace. Focus on your dreams and goals, and enjoy achievements and success. Taste them rather than compete.

Don't Worry

Most people are worried about something, but 90% of your worries not resolved. When the future is uncertain, you may worry about the future. Avoid focusing on the worst-case under adverse circumstances, as this is harmful to your health. You have learned to live for today, not tomorrow. Also, avoid worrying about what others think of you because it doesn't matter. Be your true self, rather than hiding behind the curtain wall to appease others. No matter what you do, no matter who you are, you can never please everyone. If you want some people, you will offend others, so try to be your best self. To quote "A Practical Guide to Wake Up Life": "If your happiness depends on life is a special way. Then it means that the flow of life will eventually dissolve the environment that brings you happiness, just like the tide washed away your writing on the beach."

Develop a Positive Outlook

Without a positive vision, our lives will not be happy. Follow the above suggestions and develop an optimistic attitude. It requires work and regular attention, but the reward is worth it. As I have seen in my life, even if we are not aware, everything will happen for our best interests.

Have you been fired recently? Perhaps an exciting career is waiting for you to complete your current job? By adding a positive attitude to what is happening, your life will become better. "Most of us don't want to be disturbed. We don't want any difficulty in the pursuit of Happiness. What we want is happiness is on the plate. But to find out what real happiness is, we must be willing to be disturbed, surprised, and wrong in our assumptions and fall deeply into the unknown abyss."

Be Energetic and Optimistic

Don't let adverse circumstances and grief spread or ruin your life. Whenever you feel sad, please raise your head as much as possible. It would help if you told yourself that life is full of hope, challenges, and unexpected twists and turns. We are looking for the silver lining in life. Something that we think is bad happens in life. However, when we look at it, it has some functional aspects. These are called the silver lining. E.g.: Your partner dumped you. A silver lining? You can meet many different people. The opportunity to meet someone and let them enter their hearts and souls is a significant thing.

You lost your job. Maybe you don't like your post very much. A silver lining? You now have the opportunity to find a better, more meaningful, and higher-paying position. When you think you will succeed, you fail? Life is so exciting, isn't it? A silver lining? The knowledge you gain from failure is the same or more than the knowledge gained from getting the right for the first time.

189

Reasons to Smile for Yourself

Scientists have discovered that the act of smiling makes you happier. Yes: just smile. Try it. Find one of the following reasons to smile and try:

- A stranger passed you and smiled.

- Someone did a good thing to a random stranger.

- Unexpected things happen, making you have to think about how vast and strange the world is.

- You see beautiful things in the world.

Generous

You may feel smart, thinking that winning the lottery will make you happy, but you are wrong. The money will only increase happiness at a certain level that meets your basic needs. After that, money makes you more comfortable than everyone else. However, it is compassion that makes you happy. One study found that watching people donate money to charities makes us as happy as collecting money! That means that if you can, you should see a way to sympathize. Give it back to charity, volunteer as a volunteer at your local food bank, and help sophomores complete their homework.

Learn how to forgive others. Forgiving others is the act of making the past a thing of the past. If research shows that you will be a happy person, you can find in your heart forgiveness for others, even those who are not worthy or unwilling to forgive you. Forgiving others may lower blood pressure, lower overall stress levels, and lower your heart rate, thereby making you happier.

Keep Improving

A 2007 study reported data from the UK Household Panel Survey, and the results revealed a series of exciting root causes of happiness. What makes us happy: get what we want or have what we want? Paradoxically, it does not seem to make us the most comfortable state of "marriage," but a dynamic event such as "beginning a new love. "Similarly, "getting a new job" has a far more significant impact on happiness than employment. Compared with becoming a parent, "pregnancy" has a more significant effect on happiness. Similarly, events such as "starting a new course," "passing an exam," or "buying a new house" are also very high in terms of happiness.

Conversely, events with a low relationship to happiness include the end of the relationship, loss of work, and parents' loss. What does all this mean, and what makes the British people happy? Let's take a moment to solve this problem. Positive dynamic events seem to be critical rather than static. Although this may sound superficial, if you view happiness as an "instantaneous" state, it makes sense. What can we learn from this study? If you want to pursue happiness in your life or remain positive and optimistic, please realize that there are always some happy events waiting for you. If you don't want to wait, go out and do something pleasant. As Abraham Lincoln put it: "The best way to predict the future is to create it."

- People who make you smile. Research shows that when we are with those happy people, we are the most comfortable. Hold on to those happy people and move.

- Stick to your values. What you discover is true; what you know is fair, and what you believe is all values. As time goes by, the more you respect them, the better you will feel about yourself and the people you love.

- Accept well. Look at life, assess how it works, and don't give up just because it's not perfect. When good things happen, let even small things come in.

- Imagine the best. Don't be afraid to look at what you want and see that you got it. Many people avoid this process because they do not want to be disappointed when things cannot resolve. The truth is that imagining what you want is a big part of achieving it.

- Do what you like. Maybe you can't do skydiving every day or vacation every season, but as long as you do something you like from time to time, you will find greater happiness.

- Find the purpose. Those who believe in contributing to human well-being feel better about lives. Most people want to be part of something bigger than themselves simply because it is satisfactory.

- Listen to your heart. You are the only one who knows what makes you satisfied. Your family and friends may think you are good at things that keep your boat from floating. After happiness, things may get complicated. Just be smart and keep your daily work for now.

- Push yourself, don't push others. It is easy to make people feel that others are responsible for your achievements, but the fact is that this is indeed your responsibility. Once you realize this, you can get where you want to go. No longer blame others or the whole world; you will find the answer soon.

- Willing to change. Even if you feel bad, change is one thing you can rely on. The change will happen, so develop an emergency plan and emotionally support the experience.

- Enjoy simple fun. Those who love you, precious memories, stupid jokes, warm days, and starry nights—these are the bonds that are linked together, and gifts give continuously.

- Live our "best life." For beginners, we can start with the "best life" I like. That includes being the best version of ourselves. It involves self-acceptance and no longer compares oneself to others. Living our best lives also includes not using things to measure our happiness, but focusing on feelings. Practicing mindfulness can also help us achieve satisfaction. By doing so, we can fully experience the moment of the moment and learn to keep pace with the times. According to the moment of the moment, and grasp the opportunity. When we can accept the essence of things, we become happier.

- Practice daily gratitude. Gratitude determines our attitude. When we practice gratitude, it eventually becomes second nature. We can find beauty in small things and appreciate all the things that life provides.

- Learning the art of letting go When we learn to let go, we will find a way to freedom. By learning to let go, we no longer bound by past or lingering negative emotions.

- These are other things we can do to make ourselves feel good.

- Smile. Everyone knows that smiles are contagious. If you are frustrated, force a smile and keep it smiling. If you don't want to smile, you will end up giggling because of being silly.

- Smell something that makes you happy. The sense of smell is compelling and can trigger a variety of emotions and reactions. Why not smell the road to happiness? Smell the flowers you like, inhale the aroma you want, or indulge in the food you like. When I'm down,

I smell the lavender. Not only do I love this smell, but it also has some calming and relaxing properties.

- Do what is right for others. If you cannot show a smile on your face, please smile on someone else's face. Doing good deeds usually brings that kind of joy, joy. How do you avoid smiling when you become someone for a day?

- Do things you haven't done in a while, remember the wind that blows on your face when you swing, or play baseball, or do a lot of good things, that happy cookie? Okay, get up and move! Like doing pleasant things that have never done in a while, this is not fussy. Think back to the little things that make you happy, and then explore again.

- Laugh, laugh, laugh. Smiles are contagious, as are smiles. Watch funny movies or recall some exciting things, then laugh. If you can't think of anything ridiculous, start laughing and continue thinking. You must think of something exciting or continue to laugh at yourself.

Benefits of Happiness in Life

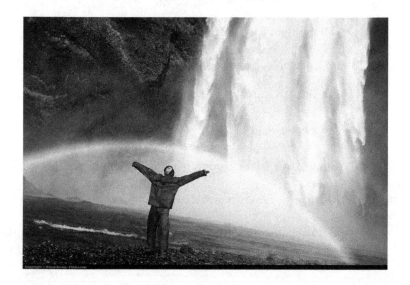

Happiness Increases Productivity

Consider a study that measures people's initial well-being and then tracks their work performance over the next 18 months. Even after controlling other factors, happy people initially paid higher, and later got better evaluations. A similar study measured the happiness level of first-year students. Nineteen years later, it predicted how high their income would be, regardless of their initial financial situation. In general, happy workers are more productive, more efficient as leaders, generate more sales, take less time off due to illness, and receive higher salaries and higher performance levels.

Happiness Improves Health

One of the most critical studies of happiness includes the diaries of 180 Catholic nuns born before 1917. Fifty years later, the researchers studied these diary entries and expressed positive emotional content for them. The results are shocking. The higher the positive level of people in their 20s, the longer these nuns live. There is a seven-year difference in life expectancy between the happiest and the happiest nuns! At any age, the nuns who use the least positive emotion words (e.g., satisfaction, appreciation, hope, love, or happiness) are twice as likely to die as the nun. She uses the most positive emotion words.

By the age of 85, 90% of the happiest quartile nuns were still alive, while only 34% were the happiest quartile. Happiness is right for your health. Other studies have shown that it can predict lower heart rate and blood pressure. It can eliminate stress, strengthen the immune system, and protect you from pain and suffering. Consider an experiment that exposed 350 adults to a common cold. Before the contact, the researchers called them six times in two weeks and asked how often they experienced nine positive emotions (for example, feeling calm, happy, or energetic).

One week after the injection of the virus, people who experienced more positive emotions in the weeks before the experiment were able to resist the infection than their unhappy peers better. They feel better, but they also reduce symptoms such as coughing, sneezing, or congestion. I found a fascinating experiment showing that the same person's immune system activity fluctuates according to their happiness. In the past two months, 30 dental students have taken pills containing harmless blood proteins from rabbits, which have produced an immune response to the human body. Participants rated their happiness by indicating whether they experienced various positive emotions that day. In the happy days, through the presence of antibodies against foreign bodies, the student's immune response is better.

Happiness Relieves Stress and Anxiety

Imagine that you have just volunteered to participate in a mood and cardiovascular responsiveness study. When you visit the laboratory, you told to sit in a comfortable chair and then connect it with a miniature sensor on your skin to measure the instantaneous changes in heart rate, blood pressure, and vasoconstriction. So far, this is a strange and unfamiliar situation, but it's no big deal. Okay, this changed the moment the researchers told you about the assignment: preparing a speech about "why you are a good friend." We will record a video of the address, and other participants will evaluate you.

Your heart beats faster. Blood pressure rises, veins, and arteries contract. In other words, you feel anxious and stressed. Next, the system will tell you that if "accidentally" shows a movie clip in preparation for a speech, it means that "computer" puts you in a "silent" state. The beginning of the movie indicates that you have got rid of the dilemma of delivering a terrible voice. A movie clip show to all participants and the real experiment was to observe how different movie clips affect stress recovery—two of the films induced positive emotions, one negative emotion, and one neutral sentiment.

The moment the movie clip began, the researchers began to track the effects of different emotions on recovery. They followed the time it took for each person's cardiovascular response to return to the baseline rest level, measured when they sat in a comfortable chair. Some hearts subside within a few seconds, while others take more than a minute to calm down. What is the difference? Participants who watched one of the frontal clips recovered the fastest from stress and anxiety. Those who saw negative or neutral editing recovered the most rapidly.

Happiness Help You Recover from Stress

Barbara Fredrickson, one of the researchers in this study, called this the "undo the effect." Generally speaking, happiness can calm down or "eliminate" stress, anxiety, depression, or adverse consequences. The next time you feel stressed, you can find something positive. Remind your family, call a friend, or watch a short movie about your favorite comedy show. If your loved one is under pressure, don't let the pressure remind them of the high risks they face. Instead, give them positive gifts. Remind them of their strengths; love their friends and family, or their upcoming activities.

Happiness Makes You Do Your Best

An experiment required four-year-old to complete a series of learning tasks, such as putting blocks of different shapes together. A group told to put these blocks together as soon as possible.

The other group also received the same instructions but was told to think about something that pleased them. Result? The children were "ready," —meaning that the researchers evoked some emotion or mind-set before the experiment— because the sense of well-being was significantly better than other children, thus completing the task faster and making fewer mistakes.

Another experiment produced even more impressive results. During the training, a medical test usually performed by doctors was based on the patient's symptoms and medical history. If you have ever watched the TV series "Maryland House," you will know what we are talking about here. In this experiment, the doctors in training divide into three groups. A group of people was happy before making a diagnosis. Ask another person to read neutral materials and give the control group no special instructions before practicing.

Happiness-based doctors ultimately make the correct diagnosis twice as fast as other people. They are also unlikely to be caught in what calls anchoring. This phenomenon occurs when the document is difficult to let go of the initial diagnosis (anchor point), even when faced with updated information that contradicts the initial diagnosis.

Investing in the brain for happiness is not only useful for children and doctors. Another study showed that students who told to think about the happiest day before taking the math exam performed better than their peers. Moreover, people who show positivity when negotiating business transactions are more effective than people who express neutral or negative emotions.

Happiness Creates Success

The association advocates a simple success/happiness model: if you work hard, you will succeed; once you have enough success, you will feel happy. Now don't even worry about happiness. First, be successful, and then happiness will follow. Once you make enough money, drive a beautiful car, own a beautiful house, and succeed in your career, you will be happy. If this is not the case, maybe you can lose the last five pounds, make more money, upgrade the wardrobe, and be satisfied. Continue to pursue success, and once you succeed, you will feel happy.

However, don't try to be happy now! If you are not successful enough, it will be in vain. First, you need to work hard and sacrifice your health and friendship; then, you will be happy automatically. Don't worry about happiness; double success. The only problem with this model? There will always be more successful in the pursuit of success. More money, more fame, more power—it will never end. After getting a promotion, you will set sail for another goal. Once this goal achieves, there will be another goal. Most of us pursue one goal after another, hoping that success is ultimately related to making the next goal. Before we knew it, life was over, and we were happier than ever.

What if we "success" and achieve success outside the world? That is the fate of addicted Hollywood stars and grumpy millionaires, not an example of prosperity and happiness. However, more importantly, the formula has been broken because it is backward. As you just learned, happiness promotes performance more than anything else. By sacrificing happiness, we limit our potential for success. Happiness brings more success than success.

Happiness Protects Your Heart

Love and happiness may not come from the heart, but they are suitable for the soul. For example, a 2005 paper found that satisfaction can predict lower heart rate and blood pressure. In this study, participants evaluated their own happiness 30 times a day and then assessed them three years later. The happiest participants initially had a lower heart rate during follow-up (six beats per minute), while the most joyful participants during the follow-up had higher blood pressure.

The study also found a link between happiness and another indicator of heart health: heart rate variability, which refers to the time interval between heartbeats and the risk of various diseases. In a 2008 study, the researchers monitored 76 patients suspected of having coronary heart disease. Even among people who may suffer from heart disease, is happiness linked to a healthy heart? It looks like this: On the day of the cardiac examination, the participant who rated himself as the happiest had a more robust heart rate variability pattern on that day.

Over time, these effects can exacerbate significant changes in heart health. In a 2010 study, investigators invited nearly 2,000 Canadians to enter the laboratory to talk about their anger and stress. Observers rated their positive emotions (happiness, happiness, excitement, enthusiasm, and satisfaction) on a scale of 1-5. Ten years later, the researchers checked with the participants to see their living conditions—and found that happy people are less likely to have coronary heart disease. Each point of positive emotion they express increases their heart disease risk by 22%.

Happiness Will Strengthen Your Immune System

Do you know a grumpy person and always get sick? That may not be accidental: research is finding a link between happiness and a more robust immune system. In an experiment in 2003, 350 adults volunteered to participate in the common cold (don't worry, they were well-compensated). Before the contact, the researchers called them six times in two weeks and asked how many nine positive emotions they had that day (such as feeling energetic, happy, and calm). After five days in the quarantine, the most active participants were less likely to catch a cold.

The same researchers also wanted to investigate why happier people might not be susceptible to illness, so in a 2006 study, they provided the hepatitis B vaccine to 81 graduate students. After receiving the first two doses, participants self-assessed these nine positive emotions. People with high positive emotions are almost twice as likely to produce top antibody responses to the vaccine, which signifies a healthy immune system. Happiness does not only seem to affect symptoms but works at the cellular level.

An earlier experiment found that the immune system activity of the same person fluctuated according to their happiness. In the past two months, 30 male dentistry students have taken pills containing harmless blood proteins from rabbits, causing human immune responses. They also assessed whether they experienced various positive emotions that day. During their happy days, the participants' immune response was better, as measured by antibodies against foreign bodies in the saliva.

Happy People Have Less Pain and Suffering

Unhappiness can be painful. A 2001 study asked members to rate their most recent positive emotional experience. Then (five weeks later) evaluate how many negative symptoms they have experienced since the survey began (such as muscle strain, dizziness, and heartburn). The person who showed the highest positive emotions at the beginning became healthier during the research process and eventually became healthier than the unhappy person. Their health has improved within five weeks (the health of the most unfortunate participants has declined), a fact that shows that the results don't just show that people in good moods rated health more than people in bad feelings high.

A 2005 study showed that positive emotions could also reduce the pain caused by disease. Women with arthritis and chronic pain evaluate themselves with positive emotions (such as interest, enthusiasm, and inspiration) for about three months each week. During the study, people with higher overall scores were less likely to experience increased pain.

Happiness Fights with Sickness

Happiness is also associated with more severe and long-term improvement, not just short-term pain and suffering. In a 2008 study of nearly 10,000 Australians, members who reported that they were satisfied or happy most of the time with life were likely to suffer from long-term health conditions (such as chronic pain and severe vision problems) two years later Reduced by 1.5 times. Another education in the same year found that females with breast cancer looked back more unhappy and optimistic than women without breast cancer before being diagnosed, suggesting that happiness and optimism may have a protective effect on preventing this disease.

As adults grow up, another condition that often causes them suffering is weakness, which is characterized by a decline in strength, endurance, and balance, putting them at risk of disability and death? In a 2004 study, more than 1,550 Mexican Americans over the age of 65 were satisfied with their self-esteem, hope, happiness, and enjoyment over the past week. After seven years, participants with higher emotional scores are less likely to become weak. Some of the same academics also found that in the next six years, happy seniors (measured by the same positive emotions) are less likely to stroke. That is especially true for men.

Happiness Extends our Lifespan

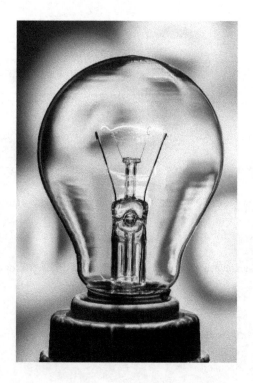

Finally, the ultimate health indicator may be longevity—especially happiness plays a role here. In the most critical study on happiness and longevity, the life expectancy of Catholic nuns is related to the positive emotions expressed in the autobiographical articles they wrote when they entered the monastery decades ago (usually in their 20s). The researchers combed these writing samples to express feelings of entertainment, satisfaction, gratitude, and love. In the end, the happiest nun looked 7 to 10 years longer than the happiest nun.

However, you don't have to be a nun to experience the life that happiness brings. In a 2011 study, nearly 4,000 British adults between the ages of 52-79 reported that they were happy, excited, and satisfied many times a day. Here, happy people are about 35% less likely to die than unhappy people in about five years. Both studies measured specific positive emotions, but overall satisfaction with life (another significant indicator of happiness) is also related to longevity. A 2010 study tracked nearly 7,000 people from Alameda County, California, for almost three decades, and found that people who were more satisfied with their lives were less likely to die during the study.

Although happiness can extend our lifespan, it cannot create miracles. There is evidence that the link between happiness and longevity does not extend to illness, or it does not extend to disease.

The 2005 meta-analysis summarized the results of other studies on health and well-being, speculating that experiencing positive emotions is helpful for longer-term diseases, but may be harmful to excellent conditions. The research cited by the authors shows that positive emotions can reduce the risk of death in patients with diabetes and AIDS. It increases the risk of death in patients with metastatic breast cancer, early melanoma, and advanced kidney disease. This increased risk may be because happier people underestimated their symptoms and did not receive the correct treatment or better care of themselves because they were too optimistic.

As the science of happiness and health matures, researchers are trying to determine the role (if any) of joy in bringing health benefits. They also attempted to distinguish the effects of different forms of happiness (including positive emotions and life satisfaction), the results of "extreme" pleasure, and other factors. For example, a new study shows that we should pay attention not only to the level of life satisfaction. But also, to the variability of life satisfaction: researchers have found that low life satisfaction (i.e., unstable happiness) caused by life fluctuations compare with death. Early death leads to death. Meet alone.

Research on the health benefits of happiness is still very young. It will take a period to number out the exact mechanism by which happiness affects health and how factors such as social relationships and exercise can adapt. But at the same time, what is certain is that happier people will also become healthier.

Happy People Are Less Ill

A Carnegie Mellon University study found that happy people are less likely to catch a cold, while depressed, nervous, or angry people are more likely to complain of severe symptoms. The authors report that happy study participants did not have a high frequency of infection, and they rarely experienced symptoms even when they were sick.

Happy People Have More Friends

Let's face it: happy people will be more enjoyable together. No one wants to spend too much time on Donald. That is why social relations are so important: warm, intimate friendships provide a stable support system. Good friends are verifying, inspiring, and inspiring. They enhance our sense of purpose and belonging, and countless studies have shown that strong social bonds are the key to a happy life. Not surprisingly, happy people will have more friends because they are stable, helpful, and helpful.

Happy People Donate More to Charities

You may have heard that generosity lights up the brain's pleasure and reward areas. When people expose to things such as art, charming faces, and cocaine; these areas light up. Science shows that it has two effects: giving others makes us happier, but happy people are unhappy. People contribute more to charity. This study shows that researchers at Harvard Business School concluded: "Happy people pay more, and then feel happier, pay more, and so on."

Happy People Will Be More Helpful

Similarly, happy people are more willing. Research shows that happy people are more likely to participate in voluntary activities, and people who do so tend to become more comfortable. (This is another indication of the circular relationship with happiness.)A happy person is a helpful person. When you are in a positive emotional state, you will be able to be better able to change the world better.

Having a Positive Attitude Will Make Life Easier

The optimistic mood can alleviate pain, sorrow, and grief. Bad things don't stop happening, as long as you have an upbeat attitude, you can respond better. Asked about the Holocaust survivor who lived for 108 years, Alice Herz-Sommer asks how to be happy after such a tragedy. She replied: "I'm looking for benefits. I know there are bad things, but I'm looking for benefits." Being able to see the positive side (even if things are tough) is also a secret to a happy life.

Have a Positive Impact on The People You Love?

Do you know the nights when your husband, wife, roommate, or child is in a bad mood? The whole house reacts to negative energy. You stand there and watch bad emotions flow from one room to another. The same thing happens with "happy energy." We influence each other. Therefore, if you want others to be happy, please express your enthusiasm when greeting them.

Happy People like More In-depth Conversations

Gossip is a dialogue between negative thinkers. Dr. Matthias Mehl reported in the Journal of Psychological Science that happy people have twice as many meaningful conversations as unhappy people.

Happy People Smile More

Ron Gut man said in a viral TED speech: "Smile sends a signal to the emotionally happy brain." It is suitable for your health—reducing stress hormones and blood pressure—and, in extending your lifespan. Other studies have found that people who smile often have higher ratings of tolerance, trustworthiness, and extroversion.

Happy People Exercise More and Eat More Healthily

You already know that exercise has countless benefits for your health. So, where does happiness come from? Research shows that when you feel happy, you are more likely to develop good habits, such as more exercise and a healthy diet, to improve your health.

Happy People are Satisfied with What They Have

You were kissing jealousy. Bye! The happiest of us know that being jealous of others is a misuse of their time. It doesn't matter if things don't last forever. When you are happy, you are less likely to be stressed because you want more, envy others, or try to keep up with Jones. Being satisfied with what you have allows you to focus on enriching your life and living a meaningful life.

CONCLUSION

Thank you for reading all this book!

Affirmations also relieve anxiety. You can alleviate the stress by watching the exciting things, try yoga, stop multitasking, do some banking, meditation, walk in nature, visualization, and try a hypnotic yourself. Focusing on positive words has power, which is certainly true when it comes to hypnosis. Within the framework of hypnosis, we almost always have to focus on the positive aspects. For Staying positive some of the techniques are: start a new day from peace- meditation, do it to others, just like you want others to do to you, agree that everything cannot be controlled, be proud of yourself, willing to see constant changes, grant yourself the right to succeed, surround yourself with decisive force, say your success is a current fact, not a plan, create visual space, determine your resistance, start a thank you diary, release your attachment to operation method, surrounded with allies, pay attention to your diet, participate in healthy fitness programs.

You should focus on positive thoughts, such as beliefs in their abilities, positive attitudes to challenges, and attempts to make the lousiest environment. Bad things will happen. Sometimes you disappointed. It does not mean that the world will attract you, nor does it mean that everyone will let you down. Instead, it would help if you looked at the situation realistically, find ways to improve it, and learn from experience.

Overweight can be symptoms of many chronic and somatic diseases such as type II diabetes mellitus, prolactinoma, polycystic ovary syndrome, early menopause, disease adrenal glands. The reason for overweight and obesity increases the consumption of food with high fats, decreases physical activity, and changes transportation methods. People want to lose weight to get rid of the diseases. Some people want to look stunning, rejoice at the reflection in the mirror and photographs, put on your clothes again, and lightness. You can lose weight by meditation as through it; you can be ready to deal with your thoughts, feelings, self-esteem, and how you perceive yourself. You will prepare to dig into the emotional triggers and past traumas that are no healthy and their relationship with food. In meditation, you can find the truth about why you always skip your daily workout or take a quick meal at night. You can explore the motivation for weight loss and why you could not achieve your weight loss goals. You can connect the dots to create a unique approach so that you maintain your weight as well as find peace with food and your body through meditation. If you are struggling with meditation, you should start can start bt trying to be more careful when preparing the meals and become more aware of all the unhealthy habits which trigger which do not serve your weight loss goal.

You have already taken a step towards your improvement.

Best wishes!

CPSIA information can be obtained
at www.ICGtesting.com
Printed in the USA
BVHW091653250521
608095BV00003B/907